MANAGING
CONTRACEPTION

2005-2007
For Your Pocket

Contraceptive
Technology
For Your Desk

Pills & NuvaRing for Extended Cycles

Robert A. Hatcher
Mimi Zieman
Carrie Cwiak
Philip D. Darney
Mitchell D. Creinin
Harriet R. Stosur

Implanon

DMPA for Endometriosis

Subcutaneous DMPA for Endometriosis

Tools for Teaching Contraception

ParaGard & Mirena

800,000
Copies in
Circulation
June 2005

Order copies @ www.managingcontraception.com

TABLE OF CONTENTS

OUR MISSION

The mission of *Bridging The Gap Foundation* is to improve reproductive health and contraceptive decision-making of women and men by providing up-to-date educational resources to the physicians, nurses and public health leaders of tomorrow.

OUR VISION

Our vision is to provide educational resources to the health care providers of tomorrow to help ensure informed choices, better service, better access to service, happier and more successful contraceptors, competent clinicians, fewer unintended pregnancies and disease prevention.

www.managingcontraception.com
Examples of questions answered on this website:

Hormones: I don't have a biological background, so it would be helpful for ◄ me to have definitions of the hormones a woman produces and the hormones present in birth control pills. How do these hormones affect the uterus? What are the differences between estrogens and progestins?

IUDs: If a patient has a distant history (8 years ago) of a carcinoma in situ ◄ on her Pap smear that was followed up and everything found to be clear after follow-up and treatment, would you recommend an IUD placement if she so desires? She has also had negative pap smears for 3-4 years in a row. She does have a distant history of PID, but is currently in a monogamous relationship. What information can you give me on IUD placement after carcinoma in situ?

Depo-Provera: What do you think about the new boxed warnings on Depo- ◄ Provera regarding bone loss and not using it greater than 2 years unless an alternative contraceptive can be found for a woman and her clinician? Should the warning change my prescribing habits? I work in college health and have a great many patients on Depo-Provera and many for more than 2 years.

NuvaRing: Some clinicians think that women will not be willing to place ◄ a foreign body into the vagina and then remove it. Yet, many clinicians have been successful introducing NuvaRing to patients and gaining their acceptance. How is NuvaRing presented to women by these clinicians? Do clinicians place a NuvaRing into the vagina of women to show them how easy it is to do this and how comfortable NurvaRing is? Do clinicians have women remove and reinsert NuvaRing for themselves?

COPYRIGHT INFORMATION

IMPORTANT DISCLAIMER

The authors remind readers that this book is intended to educate health care providers, not guide individual therapy. The authors advise a person with a particular problem to consult a primary-care clinician or a specialist in obstetrics, gynecology, or urology (depending on the problem or the contraceptive) as well as the product package insert and other references before diagnosing, managing, or treating the problem. **Under no circumstances should the reader use this handbook in lieu of or to override the judgment of the treating clinician.** The order in which diagnostic or therapeutic measures appear in this text is not necessarily the order that clinicians *should* follow in each case. The authors and staff are not liable for errors or omissions.

Eighth Edition, 2005-2007
ISBN 0-9638875-7-2
Printed in the United States of America
The Bridging the Gap Foundation

On 171 pages, we cannot possibly provide you with all the information you might want or need about contraception. Many of the questions clinicians ask are answered in the textbook *Contraceptive Technology* or in detail on our website. Visit us regularly at:

www.managingcontraception.com

A POCKET GUIDE TO

MANAGING CONTRACEPTION

2005-2007 Edition

Robert A. Hatcher, MD, MPH
Professor of Gynecology and Obstetrics
Emory University School of Medicine

Mimi Zieman, MD
Associate Professor of Gynecology and Obstetrics
Emory University School of Medicine

Carrie Cwiak, MD, MPH
Assistant Professor of Gynecology and Obstetrics
Emory University School of Medicine

Philip D. Darney, MD, MSc
Professor of Obstetrics, Gynecology and Reproductive Sciences
University of California, San Francisco
San Francisco General Hospital

Mitchell D. Creinin, MD
Professor of Obstetrics, Gynecology and Reproductive Sciences
University of Pittsburgh School of Medicine
Magee-Womens Hospital

Harriet R. Stosur, MD
Clinician in Obstetrics and Gynecology, Northwest Permanente
Portland, Oregon

Technical and Computer Support:
Anna Poyner, Max Harrell, Don Bagwell
Digital Impact Design, Inc., Cornelia, Georgia

Special Thanks: Copies of *A Pocket Guide to Managing Contraception* are being sent to all 3rd year medical students in the United States thanks to the **David and Lucile Packard Foundation**. We are extremely grateful. If you know of 3rd year medical students who have not received copies of this book, please notify us at our website **www.managingcontraception.com**.

The Bridging the Gap Foundation • Tiger, Georgia

Dear Colleagues and Friends:

Managing Contraception has always been a practical and useful source of clinical information for students, residents, and providers who deal with reproductive health issues. Collaboration in education is the focus of this year's eighth edition. We have dedicated the handbook to Dr. Denise Jamieson and Dr. Roger Rochat, two clinicians that have dedicated countless hours to students and residents working to achieve their own educational goals. In addition, our interactive learning tool has been updated for use with this edition of *Managing Contraception*. This interactive tool uses problem-based learning to incourage active student participation in their learning of all the available methods of contraception. The list of questions, as well as suggestions for use of the learning tool, can be found on the following pages (ii-v). Educators can easity adopt this tool for use in their own setting; our goal is to make it as easy as possible to teach your students and colleagues up-to-date contraceptive information and to familiarize them to the potential clinical uses of the handbook.

The interactive teaching tool is also available in power point format on CD-ROM. The power point slides contain photos of all available contraceptive methods and are an effective complement to theinteractive session. The CD-ROM can be ordered through our website: www.managingcontraception.com. When tested among third year medical students, this interactive teaching tool, combined with the slide set, resulted in a significant gain in knowledge and above-average satisfaction scores, equal to that of a traditional lecture.

As in previous years, this edition of *Managing Contraception* will be provided to all U.S. medical students and residents in obstetrics and gynecology and family medicine programs. This is possible due to the generosity of the David and Lucille Packard Foundation. Nurses, nursing students and advanced care providers have also received copies of *Managing Contraception*. In total, 800,000 copies of the handbook are in circulation!

Managing Contraception has been designed as a pocket-sized handbook in order to provide an immediate source of clinical information. In these pages, we cannot possibly cover all of the available information on contraception. *Contraceptive Technology* is a textbook that is a comprehensive reference for your questions about reproductive health issues, contraceptive management, sexually transmitted infections, and sexuality issues. The eighteenth revised edition of the text was published in 2004, and is available through the website in soft-cover, CD-ROM, and PDA formats.

For our dedicated *Managing Contraception* users, find out what's new in this edition with a quick flip through the handbook. Remember, just look for the bold arrows!

We hope you enjoy the new handbook and educational tool. Please feel free to send us your questions/comments about either the handbook or interactive tool through the website: www.managingcontraception.com.

Carrie Cwiak, MD, MPH
Assistant Professor
Department of Gynecology and Obstetrics
Emory University School of Medicine
Atlanta, Georgia

Alison Edelman, MD, MPH
Assistant Professor
Department of Obstetrics and Gynecology
Oregon Health and Sciences University
Portland, Oregon

HOW TO USE THE INTERACTIVE LECTURE

• Medical students can receive the handbook, ***Managing Contraception*** (2005-2007 Edition), and a handout with the self-learning questions at the beginning of their OB/GYN or Family Practice clinical clerkship. You may copy the questions directly from this book.

• Students in other disciplines (nursing, public health, etc.) can receive the handbook and questions at the beginning of any clinical rotation or semester in which reproductive health issues will be discussed.

• The lecture can be used within the context of an OB/GYN or other residency program to teach residents about contraception in an interactive, case-based format.

• The lecture can be presented as an interactive inservice to the reproductive health providers (MD's, NP's, PA's) in your clinic or department. The lecture then also serves as an introduction to the potential uses of ***Managing Contraception*** for providers in their day-to-day clinical activities.

• Equally divide the self-learning questions between the students/providers in each rotation or class. Students should have their questions prepared in time for the lecture. Each question takes approximately 5 minutes to answer. All answers can be found in the handbook. The page numbers that accompany each question can direct students to the answers.

• Become familiar with the lecture and the topic. The CD-rom, "Teaching Contraception: An Interactive Lecture Using ***Managing Contraception***" contains powerpoint slides that can accompany the lecture. The slides contain photos of all the methods. The CD-rom also provides supplemental information, page numbers, and answers in the 'NOTES' section of the lecture. To order the CD, please contact Bridging the Gap at (706) 265-7435 or **www.managingcontraception.com**.

• The lecture works best when it is as interactive as possible – have the students help present the lecture! Your input is meant to enhance each student's answer and to initiate discussion about their assigned question. The powerpoint lecture on CD-rom can help with this task as well.

• If you desire to give the lecture in one session, it takes approximately 2 hours to present. The lecture can easily be split into 3 sessions: Combined (Estrogen-Containing) Contraceptives, Progestin-Only Contraceptives, and Hormone-Free Contraceptives.

• Have fun with it! Bring examples of different birth control methods to show, props, etc.

Combined (Estrogen-Containing) Contraceptives:

1. Give three examples of ways of **starting birth control pills** other than on Sunday from among the many in Table 26.2. Which of these do you think is easiest to explain? Pages 109-110, 114

2. What is the take home message about **how to choose or prescribe a pill**? Can a woman who is able to use estrogen be prescribed **any of the sub-50 mcg pills**? What is the difference between a monophasic and a multiphasic pill? Pages 101, 106, 115

3. Your patient is starting to take combined pills. You want to quickly teach her what to watch out for. Use the letters **ACHES** to remind her what to watch out for. Pages A-29, 104, bottom of page 112

4. A woman stopped taking her combined oral contraceptive, Alesse, 2 months ago and had unprotected sex last night. She would like to use her Alesse for **emergency contraception** now. How would you instruct her to use this pill as an emergency contraceptive? What is a more effective EC for her? Pages 77, 79, 82-83, 86, A-30

5. A 26-year-old is using the weekly **Evra patch** method of contraception and just realized that she has left her patch on for 10 days. How effective is the patch in the first year with perfect use? Is it still effective now on day 10? How long can her patch-free interval be? Pages 39, 119, 121

6. A 30-year-old likes the menstrual regularity she gets with her combined pills, but forgets to take them everyday. She wants to use the vaginal **Nuva ring** for contraception. Instruct her in its use. Specifically: How long does she leave it in? How long does she wait before inserting a new ring? Should she remove it during intercourse? If she does, how long can she leave it out? Pages 121-123

7. Discuss the contraceptive options for a woman **24 hours postpartum** if she is likely to have intercourse before the postpartum visit (despite medical instructions)? Pages 29, 92

8. You are seeing a woman in your office with **a blood pressure of 165/105**. What methods of contraception should you be cautious in prescribing? What methods could she use if her blood pressure were well controlled? Pages A-3, 106, 131

Progestin-Only Contraceptives

9. A woman had unprotected sex 1.5 days ago and is considering **emergency contraceptive pills**. She asks you: How do they work? Will they cause an abortion? How soon after unprotected sex do I need to take them? Will they protect me for the rest of my cycle? Please answer her questions. Pages 77, 79-80, 82, 86

10. A 19 year-old woman recently received a **Depo-Provera** shot and is concerned about **irregular bleeding**. How would you counsel her about this? What if she had amenorrhea? Pages 128, 132-134

11. You see a woman who has **gained 25 pounds** in the last 18 months. She believes it is related to her Depo-Provera. How do you counsel her? In 60 seconds give her some suggestions. Pages 129, 132, 134

12. What are 5 noncontraceptive advantages of **Mirena,** the levonorgestrel intrauterine contraceptive? What is the most important disadvantage of Mirena? Page 95-96

13. What advice do you give to a 28 year-old using **progestin-only pills** for contraception if she is also **taking carbamazepine** for seizures? What other medications should you ask about? Is there a better method for her? Pages 125-126, 128, A-8

14. A 40 year-old wants to use oral contraceptives but is a **smoker.** What kind of oral contraceptives should you recommend? What are the disadvantages of these pills? Pages 124-125, A-3

15. Your 30 year-old patient used **Norplant** implants in the past and is asking if there is an implant available now that she can use. For how many years is this implant effective? How many capsules are there? Pages 137-138.

16. A 17 year-old nulligravid teenager has been using Depo-Provera for the last 2 years. You have just diagnosed her with **PID.** If she still wants to use Depo-Provera in the future, how can she protect herself from infection? How would you teach her to use the male condom, for example? Pages 58-59, 129

Non-Hormonal Contraceptives

17. A 30 year-old woman is considering a **Copper IUD** and asks: How does it work? Do IUD's cause an abortion? How long are they effective? Do they cause ectopic pregnancies or future infertility? Please answer her questions. Pages 88-89

18. A woman wants to have sex with her boyfriend but he will not wear a condom because he says he is, **"allergic to latex."** What advice can you give her? What are the other types of condoms? Pages 56-59

19. What issues should you counsel patients about before tubal sterilization? How effective are the different **tubal sterilization** methods? Pages 140-145

20. A 34 year-old man has just gotten a **vasectomy.** When can his partner stop using her contraceptive method? Pages 147-148

21. An 19 year-old college student is using **spermicides** as her only method of contraception. She asks you: How effective are spermicides in protecting against pregnancy? Do spermicides affect her risk of acquiring HIV and other STI's? What other method(s) would you suggest? Pages 39, 72-73

22. What are some of the advantages of the **Reality female condom** when compared to the male condom? What are some of the disadvantages? Pages 56-57, 63-64

23. A 16 year-old girl was told by her boyfriend that the **withdrawal** method of birth control is just as effective as not having sex at all. What can you advise her about the effectiveness of the withdrawal method for contraception? For what else would she be at risk? Pages 39, 75-76

24. A 36 year-old is using a latex **diaphragm** for birth control as well as a lubricant for vaginal dryness. What lubricants or creams should she avoid? What other birth control methods can be affected by these products? Pages 61, 68, 71

25. A 30-year old is curious about the **cervical cap** and wants to know: In what ways is the cap different from the diaphragm? In what ways is it the same? Pages 66-68, 69-71

26. Your patient has just learned that she has a **positive pregnancy test**. What are her options? If she decides to terminate the pregnancy, what are her 2 options? What are the relative advantages of each one? Pages 28, 31

27. Professor John Guillebaud strongly suggests using **fertility awareness in a very limited manner**. How effective are the different fertility awareness methods? Pages 39, 51-52

28. A 14 year-old plans to continue **abstinence** as her contraceptive method. What are your instructions to her? What can you provide for her before she leaves your office? Pages 42-44

29. Name the 3 conditions necessary for the **Lactational Amenorrhea Method** to be an effective contraceptive method. Pages 45-47

We dedicate this edition of **Managing Contraception** *to*
Dr. Denise Jamieson *and* **Dr. Roger Rochat**

When a research paper or thesis is required before an individual successfully completes a step in his or her education, the person who helps prepare this paper is truly a friend. **Roger Rochat** helps students at Emory's Rollins School of Public Health. Over the past four years, Roger has helped 44 students with their theses or dissertations. Here are several examples:

Mignone, Laurie: A global analysis of the inverse association of national contraceptive prevalence and maternal mortality rates. (2003)

Gaddis, Janelle: Estimates of unmet need for contraception, State of Georgia, 1996 (2004, in progress)

Veysset, Elodie: A history of sterilization in the United States (PhD Project in Women's Studies, 2001)

Tuteja, Ritu (Epidemiology): Intention status and other predictors of abortion among 3218 women, Republic of Georgia, 1995-1999 (summer 2004)

Finch, Rabiah: Men's involvement in abortion decisions in Atlanta, Georgia (2004)

Roger says he is inspired by the following words: *Our students are everything. Without students we are nothing.* Often, Roger travels to the country where his International Health students are working. His students have worked on topics in 18 countries. He has received awards at Emory for his excellence as a teacher. In past years, Roger was an Epidemic Intelligence Service Officer at the CDC and became Chief of The Division of Reproductive Health at the CDC.

Denise Jamieson's career has also included work at the CDC and at Emory. Each resident in The Department of Gynecology and Obstetrics at Emory must present to his or her peers and the faculty the results of a formal research project. This task must be completed during the very time consuming and often stressful process of learning to be a proficient physician in a complex field. In addition to helping residents understand the literature of their field through the department's journal club, below are several of the resident research projects Denise has participated in:

Ian Tilley. Medical care after sexual assault

Jennifer Franz. Outcomes of GYN surgery in HIV positive women compared to seronegative women (with Drs. Cyril Spann and Hugh Randall)

Fatu Forna. Pregnancy outcomes in foreign born women (with Dr. Michael Lindsay)

Jansvant Adusumalli. Detection of Hepatitis C through identification of risk factors

Sarah Fergerson. Diagnosing postpartum depression - can we do better? (with Dr. Michael Lindsay)

Phoebe Sun. Evaluation of fetal anomalies and termination of pregnancy. (with Dr. Denise Raynor)

Claire Parker. Methotrexate in ectopic pregnancy: predictors of rupture

Phoebe Mou. Sickle cell disease and adverse outcomes in pregnancy. (with Dr. Denise Raynor)

These two physicians have helped their students in their hour of need and, in the process, they have increased our understanding of contraceptives, HIV and reproductive health. We thank you Denise and Roger.

Many have contributed their sensitivity, time, graphics and layout skills, financial support, friendship, encouragement, patience and love in the creation of this *Pocket Guide to Managing Contraception*. This book has been a labor of love. We have tried to condense our thoughts into a format that clinicians and counselors can carry in their pockets. Gems have come to us from many corners of the world. We thank all contributors, including:

- **Jeffrey Allen**, superb, caring breast radiologist at Piedmont Hospital in Atlanta and contributing artist to MC
- **Marcus Arevalo**, Georgetown University researcher and leader in the study of fertility awareness methods
- **Kaea Beresford**, Gyn-Ob resident at Emory University; now in practice in Colorado
- **Stephen F. Brandt**, resident in internal medicine; has deep reservoirs of concern and caring and great attention to detail
- **Rachel Blankstein Breman**, author of pilot edition of *MC*
- **Sharon L. Camp**, immediate past-president, Women's Capital Corporation, the company that brought PLAN B to the United States; currently CEO of Alan Guttmacher Institute
- **Martha Campbell**, international FP consultant. She and the David and Lucile Packard Foundation made *MC* possible
- **Willard Cates**, president, Family Health International, researcher in contraception, STIs and HIV, and author of *Contraceptive Technology*; cheerleader!
- **Camaryn Chrisman,** medical student at Wake Forest, author of articles on WHO Medical Eligibility Criteria. Ob/Gyn resident, Ann Arbor, Michigan
- **Sarah Clark** and staff in the Population Program at the David and Lucile Packard Foundation. Their support of this book from the very start made this effort a reality
- **Kathryn M. Curtis**, Women's Health and Fertility Branch, CDC; author of articles on WHO Medical Eligibility Criteria
- **Anne Lange-Dunlop**, researcher on fertility awareness methods. Family practice faculty, Emory University School of Medicine
- **Alison Edelman**, Assistant professor, Department of Obstetrics and Gynecology, Oregon Health and Sciences University. See *Dear Colleagues & Friends* p. i
- **Michelle Fox**, Assistant professor of Ob/Gyn at Maryland
- **Erica Frank**, preventionist, environmentalist and associate professor of family and preventive medicine and anatomy at Emory University
- **Felicia Guest**, AIDS educator, wise observer and an author of *Contraceptive Technology*
- **John Guillebaud**, professor of family planning and reproductive health at University College London Hospitals and medical director of the Margaret Pyke Center for Study and Training in Family Planning. We thank John for permission to use information from *Contraception Today* (Martin Dunitz Ltd.), London, in *MC*
- **Peter Hatcher**, family practice physician, Multnomah County HD, Portland, Oregon; lover of gardening, photography, his family and dogs and a loyal friend
- **Jennifer Hayes**, Emory family planning fellow researching post-placental IUD insertion ◄
- **Andrew Kaunitz**, professor and assistant chair, OB/GYN department, University of Florida; Health Sciences Center, Jacksonville, Florida
- **Maxine Keel**, administrative assistant at the Emory University Family Planning Program, dreamer, inspiration and friend

- **Karla Maguire**, Virginia Commonwealth University School of Medicine, wrote ←
  Male Reproductive Health chapter 7 in *MC*
- **Lisa A. Maniscalco**, (LAM!) whose initials tell you the chapter she contributed to!
- **Missy Nasser**, nurse midwifery student at Emory
- **Anita L. Nelson**, M.D., Professor of Obstetrics and Gynecology at David Geffen School
  of Medicine at UCLA Harbor-UCLA Medical Center. Author of first five editions of *MC*
- **Betsy Patterson**, medical student at Case Western Reserve entering obstetrics and gynecology
- **Bert Peterson**, contraceptive research leader at the CDC in Atlanta and at the WHO ←
  in Geneva. Now at UNC, Chapel Hill in the School of Public Health
- **Erika Pluhar**, author of *A Personal Guide to Managing Contraception*, *SE101*
  Dissertation in human sexuality on mother/daughter communication
- **Malcolm Potts**, perhaps the most creative force in the field of family planning, human
  sexuality and reproductive health. Students at U.C. Berkeley love him
- **Dian "Tossy" Hitt Sanders**, resident in Gynecology and Obstetrics at Emory University
- **Sharon Schnare**, dreamer, nurse practitioner and nurse midwife consultant and trainer in
  Seattle; remarkable teacher
- **Cyril Spann**, Professor of Gynecology and Obstetrics, Emory University; beloved teacher ←
- **Felicia Stewart**, Adjunct Professor of Obstetrics and Gynecology at the University of
  California in San Francisco; strong believer that both the disadvantages and advantages of
  each method need to be aired. Extensive help on the NuvaRing chapter
- **Stephanie B. Teal**, Assistant Professor in the Ob/Gyn department at University of Colorado
- **Ian Tilley**, positive, constructive resident in Gynecology and Obstetrics at Emory University
- **Delores Thomas**, administrator, manager, writer at Women Health Care Nurse Practitioner
  Program. Harbor - UCLA
- **Andrea Tone**, historian in the Department of History, Technology and Society at Georgia
  Tech, Atlanta; specializing in the history of contraception
- **James Trussell**, an author of *Contraceptive Technology* who developed the failure rates
  used throughout *MC*; champion of emergency contraception
- **Marcel Vekemans**, a family planning specialist from Belgium working at INTRAH whose
  attention to detail improved this book so much
- **Jane Wamsher**, nurse practitioner at Grady Memorial Hospital in Atlanta; provided
  practical protocols and creative techniques for using book to teach
- **Lee Warner**, MPH, PhD, CDC researcher working on STDs and HIV; so much help on the
  condom chapters
- **Kim Workowski**, CDC researcher on STDs and HIV; so much help on 2002 update of CDC
  STD Guidelines
- **Susan Wysocki**, strong public advocate for excellent women's health services

ABBREVIATIONS USED IN THIS BOOK

ACOG	American College of Obstetricians & Gynecologists		**EE**	Ethinyl estradiol
AIDS	Acquired immunodeficiency syndrome		**EPA**	Environmental Protection Agency
			EPT	Estrogen-progestin therapy
AMA	American Medical Association		**ERT**	Estrogen replacement therapy
ASAP	As soon as possible		**ET**	Estrogen therapy
BBT	Basal body temperature		**FAM**	Fertility awareness methods
BCA	Bichloroacetic acid		**FDA**	Food and Drug Administration
BP	Blood pressure		**FH**	Family History
BTB	Breakthrough bleeding		**FSH**	Follicle stimulating hormone
BTL	Bilateral tubal ligation		**GAPS**	Guidelines for Adolescent Preventive Services
BV	Bacterial vaginosis			
CA	Cancer (if not California)		**GC**	Gonococcus/gonorrhea
CDC	Centers for Disease Control and Prevention		**GI**	Gastrointestinal
			GnRH	Gonadotrophin-releasing hormone
COCs	Combined oral contraceptives (estrogen & progestin)			
			HBsAg	Hepatitis B surface antigen
CMV	Cytomegalovirus		**HAV**	Hepatitis A virus
CT	Chlamydia trachomatis		**HBV**	Hepatitis B virus
CVD	Cardiovascular disease		**HCG**	Human chorionic gonadotrophin
D & C	Dilation and curettage			
D & E	Dilation and evacuation		**HCV**	Hepatitis C virus
DCBE	Double contrast barium enema		**HDL**	High density lipoprotein
DMPA	Depot-medroxyprogesterone acetate (Depo-Provera)		**HIV**	Human immunodeficiency virus
			HPV	Human papillomavirus
DUB	Dysfunctional uterine bleeding		**HRT**	Hormone replacement therapy (estrogen & progestin)
DVT	Deep vein thrombosis			
E	Estrogen		**HSV**	Herpes simplex virus (I or II)
EC	Emergency contraception		**HT**	Hormone therapy (estrogen & progestin post-menopausally)
ECPs	Emergency contraceptive pills ("morning-after pills")			
			IM	Intramuscular
ED	Erectile dysfunction		**IPPF**	International Planned Parenthood Federation
E$_2$	Estradiol			
			IUC	Intrauterine contraceptive
ix			**IUD**	Intrauterine device

IUP	Intrauterine pregnancy	**PLISSIT**	Permission giving
IUS	Intrauterine system		Limited information
IV	Intravenous		Simple suggestions
KOH	Potassium hydroxide		Intensive
LAM	Lactational amenorrhea method		Therapy
LDL	Low-density lipoprotein	**PMDD**	Premenstrual dysphoric disorder
LGV	Lymphogranuloma venereum	**PMS**	Premenstrual syndrome
LH	Luteinizing hormone	**po**	Latin: "per os"; orally, by mouth
LMP	Last menstrual period	**POCs**	Progestin-only contraceptives
LNG	Levonorgestrel	**POP**	Progestin-only pill (minipill)
MI	Myocardial infarction	**PP**	Postpartum
MIS	Misoprostol	**PPFA**	Planned Parenthood
MMPI	Minnesota Multiphasic		Federation of America
	Personality Inventory	**PRN**	As needed
MMR	Mumps Measles Rubella	**qid**	Four times a day
MMWR	Mortality and Morbidity	**RR**	Relative risk
	Weekly Report	**Rx**	Prescription
MPA	Medroxyprogesterone acetate	**SAB**	Spontaneous abortion
MTX	Methotrexate	**SHBG**	Sex hormone binding globulin
MVA	Manual vacuum aspiration	**SPT**	Spotting
N-9	Nonoxynol-9	**SSRI**	Selective Serotonin
NFP	Natural family planning		Reuptake Inhibitors
NSAID	Nonsteroidal anti-	**STD**	Sexually transmitted disease
	inflammatory drug	**STI**	Sexually transmitted infection
OA	Overeaters Anonymous	**Sx**	Symptoms
OB/GYN	Obstetrics & Gynecology	**TAB**	Therapeutic abortion /
OC	Oral contraceptive		elective abortion
OR	Operating Room	**TB**	Tuberculosis
P	Progesterone or progestin	**TCA**	Trichloroacetic acid
Pap	Papanicolaou	**TSS**	Toxic shock syndrome
PCOS	Polycystic ovarian syndrome	**URI**	Upper respiratory infection
PE	Pulmonary embolism	**UTI**	Urinary tract infection
PET	Polyesther (fibers)	**VTE**	Venous thromboembolism
PG	Prostaglandin	**VVC**	Vulvovaginal candidiasis
pH	Hydrogen ion concentration	**WHO**	World Health Organization
PID	Pelvic inflammatory disease	**ZDV**	Zidovudine

1. Carry it with you. Arrows are a simple way for you to find the new information in this edition: ➤ or ◀

2. Chapter 31 is taken directly from the most recent CDC recommended guidelines for the treatment of STIs. STIs alphabetized on page 152.

3. Color photos of pills will help you to determine the pill your patient is/was on (A18 - A30)

4. The pages on the menstrual cycle concisely explain a very complicated series of events. Study pages 1-4 over and over again. Favorite subjects for exams!

5. Algorithms throughout book; several that might help you are on the following pages:
   • Page 115: Choosing a pill
   • Page 116: What to do about breakthrough bleeding or spotting on pills

6. If you know the page number for the 2003-2004 edition, the information in your 2005-2007 book is likely to be on *approximately* the same page.

7. Using the back cover to find a topic is much easier than going to the index.

8. **If the print is too small, go to www. managingcontraception.com and print out pages 8" x 11", put 3-hole punches into your large-print edition, and use this larger-print edition.**

IMPORTANT CONTACTS

TOPIC	ORGANIZATION	PHONE NUMBER	WEBSITE ◀
Abortion	Abortion Hotline (NAF)	(202) 667-5881	www.prochoice.org ◀
Abuse/Rape	National Domestic Violence Hotline	(312) 663-3520	
		800-799-SAFE	www.ndvh.org
Adoption	Adopt a Special Kid-America	888-680-7349	www.adoptaspecialkid.org
	Adoptive Families of America	800-372-3300	www.adoptivefamilies.org
Breastfeeding	La Leche League	800-LA-LECHE	www.lalecheleague.org
Contraception	Planned Parenthood Federation of America	800-230-PLAN	www.ppfa.org
	Family Health International	(919) 544-7040	www.fhi.org ◀
	World Health Organization	011-41-22-791-21-11	www.who.int ◀
	Bridging the Gap Communications	(706) 265-7435	www.managingcontraception.com ◀
	Assoc. of Reproductive Health Professionals (ARHP)	(202) 466-3825	www.arhp.org ◀
Counseling	Depression and Bipolar Support Alliance	800-826-3632	www.ndmda.org
Emergency contraception	Emergency Contraception Information	888-NOT-2-LATE	not-2-late.com
HIV/AIDS	Ntl. HIV/AIDS Clinicians' Consultation Center		www.ucsf.edu/hivcntr
	Post-Exposure Prophylaxic Hotline (PEP)	888-HIV-4911	
Pregnancy	Lamaze International	800-368-4404	www.lamaze.org
	Depression After Delivery	800-944-4773	depressionafterdelivery.com
STIs	CDC Sexually Transmitted Disease Hotline	800-342-AIDS	cdc.gov/nchstp/dstd/dstdp.html

SEVERAL KEY POINTS ON MENSTRUAL PHYSIOLOGY:

- *What initiates menses (and the next cycle)* is atrophy of the corpus luteum on or about day 25 of a typical 28 day cycle. This atrophy is initiated by a decline in LH release from the anterior pituitary gland and results in a fall in serum estrogen (E) and progesterone (P) levels. Without hormonal support, the endometrium sloughs. This drop in hormonal levels is also detected by the hypothalamus and pituitary, and FSH levels increase to stimulate follicles for the next cycle (Fig. 1.1 and 1.2).

- *Anovulation in women NOT on birth control pills leads to prolonged cycles, oligomenorrhea or amenorrhea or to irregular bleeding.* The absence of progesterone in anovulatory women *not* on pills places these women at risk for endometrial hyperplasia and cancer. Recovery of ovarian function and return of ovulation has been demonstrated in women with functional hypothalamic amenorrhea who have been treated with cognitive behaviorial therapy designed to improve coping skills for circumstances and moods that exacerbate stress *[Berga-2003]*. Similar results have also been achieved in women treated with hypnotherapy *[Tschugguel-2003]*

- *The two-cell, two gonadotrophin theory:* At the very beginning of the cycle, the outer theca cells can only be stimulated by LH and produce androgens (testosterone and androstenedione) and the inner granulosa cells can only be stimulated by FSH. Androgens diffuse toward the inner layer *granulosa* cells where they are converted into estradiol (E2) by FSH-stimulated aromatase (see Figure 1.3).

- In a developing follicle, *low androgen levels* not only serve as the substrate for FSH-induced aromatization, but also <u>stimulate</u> aromatase activity. On the other hand, *high levels of androgens* (an "androgen-rich" environment as in some women with polycystic ovaries) lead to <u>inhibition</u> of aromatase activity and to follicular atresia.

- Each woman is born with 1-2 million follicles, most of which undergo atresia before puberty. Only about 10-20 follicles each month are recruited by rising FSH levels. The recruitment actually occurs during the late luteal phase of the preceeding cycle. Of those 10-20 follicles, usually only one dominant follicle ovulates. The number of follicles stimulated each month depends on the number of follicles left in the residual pool.

- FSH levels are low before ovulation as a result of negative feedback on FSH of E2 and inhibin B. The dominant follicle "escapes" the effects of falling FSH levels before ovulation, because it has more granulosa cells, more FSH receptors on each of its granulosa cells, and increased blood flow. Cut off from adequate FSH stimulation, the other nondominant follicles undergo atresia.

- When E2 production is sustained at sufficient levels (about 200 pg/ml) for more than 50 hours, negative feedback of E2 on LH reverses to positive feedback. The LH surge occurs, and about 12 hours later an oocyte is extruded.

- About 50,000 granulosa cells form the corpus luteum. Some granulosa cells continue to produce E2 and inhibins but many join the outer layers of theca cells to produce progesterone (P). Inhibin selectively suppresses FSH, not LH. The highest levels of inhibin are during the mid-luteal phase (primarily inhibin A now), causing FSH levels to be the lowest in the mid-luteal phase. At the end of the cycle (10-14 days after ovulation) if the corpus luteum is not rescued by HCG produced by the implanted trophoblast (pregnancy), the corpus luteum will undergo programmed atresia. Falling E2, P, and inhibin levels induce the release of FSH to initiate another cycle.

1

Figure 1.1 Menstrual cycle events – Idealized 28 Day Cycle

[Hatcher RA, et al. *Contraceptive Technology*. 16th ed. New York: Irvington, 1994:41]

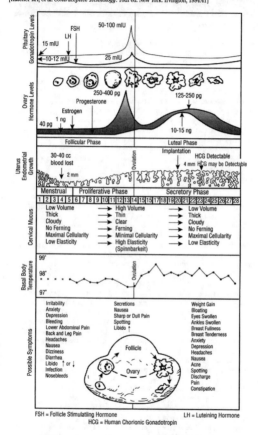

FSH = Follicle Stimulatiing Hormone
HCG = Human Chorionic Gonadotropin
LH = Luteining Hormone

Figure 1.2 Regulation of the menstrual cycle
[Hatcher RA, et al. *Contraceptive Technology*. 16th ed. New York: Irvington, 1994:40]

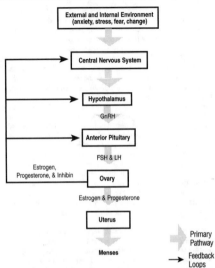

Primary hormone pathways (⇒) in the reproductive system are modulated by both negative and positive feedback loops (→). Prostaglandins, secreted by the ovary and by uterine endometrial cells, also play a role in ovulation, and may modulate hypothalamic function as well.

Figure 1.3 The two-cell, two gonadotrophin theory

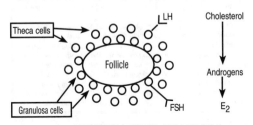

Is Menstruation Obsolete? Who Needs a Period?

The extended or continuous use of pills causes women to have fewer "pill periods". Most, but not all, women like this *[Ropes-2002]*. Decreased periods or no periods at all is important to discuss with women considering use of Seasonale pills, Depo-Provera injections, the Mirena IUD or the implant, Implanon. A 2003 gallop poll found that 99% of female gynecologists consider menstrual suppression safe. ⬅

What is "natural" — 50, 150, or 450 menstrual periods in a woman's lifetime?
In **prehistoric times** women had **50** menstrual cycles or fewer. In **Colonial America**, when women were having an average of 8 babies and nursing each baby for 2-3 years, women averaged **150** menstrual periods per lifetime. **Currently** in America women average **450-480** menstrual cycles per lifetime. *[Segal, 2001]*

Some women find regular menses reassuring, positive, "natural" or important evidence that they are still capable of reproducing. Most women regularly experiencing inconvenience, messiness, blood loss, painful menses, cyclic migraine, depression, and/or breast tenderness, would be happier having periods less often, or not at all (see discussion of extended use of COCs on page 107). ⬅

Clinicians must know how the menstrual cycle changes caused by a specific contraceptive may affect a patient coming to them for contraceptive advice. Close to half of all visits to gynecology clinicians are for difficulties women experience at the time of their menses. *[Segal, 2001]* Women with undesirable symptoms associated with their menses may benefit from contraceptives that alter the likelihood of ovulation, the amount of blood lost each month, or the extent of menstrual cramping and pain. In some instances, women may benefit from contraceptives that completely eliminate monthly periods. This is particularly likely to be true for women with any of the following cyclic symptoms: PMS, endometriosis, dysmenorrhea, depression, headaches, seizures, nausea, vomiting, breast enlargement or tenderness or very heavy bleeding. Unfortunately, few women are aware of the noncontraceptive benefits of contraceptives. *[Peipert, 1993]*

Clearly some women choose contraceptives to gain relief from symptoms related to their menstrual cycles. Others discontinue them due to undesirable effects on the patterns of their menses. In the pages ahead, the advantages and disadvantages of each contraceptive related to the menstrual cycle are described. Given the importance of the menstrual cycle to women, the sections on the effects of contraceptives on menses are very important.

A provocative book by Coutinho and Segal raises the question: *Is Menstruation Obsolete? [Coutinho, 1999]* These two individuals played pivotal roles in the research leading to the approval of a number of our current contraceptives. Here is a comment on their book:

Kate Miller, MPH, of the University of Pennsylvania states: *One of the difficulties of regular menstruation is the usual assembly of monthly symptoms - cramps, headache, fatigue, irritability - which are often dismissed as part of "the curse" that women must simply endure. Since women tolerate these symptoms so regularly, they may not automatically include them in the "risks" of monthly menstruation. The reader is encouraged to recognize what may have previously gone unnoticed: that this monthly discomfort is simply not obligatory. In fact, it can be a startling exercise for a woman to imagine her life without the hassles and ailments of regular menstruation. This is a message whose time has come.*

CHAPTER 2

Recommended Screening/Risk Assessment by Age**

AGES 13-18 YEARS

SCREENING

History
- Reason for visit
- Health status: medical, surgical, family
- Dietary/nutrition assessment
- Physical activity
- Use of complementary and alternative medicine
- Tobacco, alcohol, other drug use
- Abuse/neglect
- Sexual practices

Physical Examination
- Height and Weight
- Blood pressure
- Secondary sexual characteristics (Tanner staging)
- Pelvic examination (when indicated by the medical history) and skin*

LABORATORY TESTS

Periodic
- Cervical cytology (annually beginning at approximately 3 years after initiation of sexual intercourse)

High-Risk Groups *
- Hemoglobin level assessment
- Bacteriuria testing
- Sexually transmitted disease testing
- Human immunodeficiency virus (HIV) testing
- Genetic testing/counseling
- Rubella titer assessment
- Tuberculosis skin testing
- Lipid profile assessment
- Fasting glucose testing
- Hepatitis C virus testing
- Colorectal cancer screening+

EVALUATION AND COUNSELING

Sexuality
- Development
- High-risk behaviors
- Preventing unwanted/unintended pregnancy
  Postponing sexual involvement
  Contraceptive options, including emergency contraception
- Sexually transmitted diseases
  Partner selection
  Barrier protection

Fitness and Nutrition
- Dietary/nutritional assessment (including eating disorders)
- Exercise: discussion of program

- Folic acid supplementation (0.4 mg/d)
- Calcium intake

Psychosocial Evaluation
- Interpersonal/family relationships
- Sexual identity
- Personal goal development
- Behavioral/learning disorders
- Abuse/neglect
- Satisfactory school experience
- Peer relationships

Cardiovascular Risk Factors
- Family history
- Hypertension
- Dyslipidemia or obesity
- Diabetes mellitus

Health/Risk Behaviors
- Hygiene (including dental); fluoride supplementation
- Injury prevention
  - Safety belts and helmets
  - Recreational hazards/firearms
  - Hearing
  - Occupational hazards
  - School hazards
  - Exercise and sports involvement
- Skin exposure to ultraviolet rays
- Suicide: depressive symptoms
- Tobacco, alcohol, other drug use

IMMUNIZATIONS

Periodic
- Tetanus-diphtheria booster (once between ages 11 and 16 years)
- Hepatitis B virus vaccine (one series for those not previously immunized)

High-Risk Groups *
- Influenza vaccine
- Hepatitis A virus vaccine
- Pneumococcal vaccine
- Measles, mumps, rubella vaccine
- Varicella vaccine

Leading Causes of Death**:
- Accidents
- Malignant neoplasms
- Homicide
- Suicide
- Diseases of the heart
- Congenital anomalies

*Only for those with a family history of familial adenomatous polyposis or 8 years after the start of pancolitis. For a more detailed discussion of colorectal cancer screening, see Smith RA, von Eschenbach AC, Wender R, Levin B, Byers T, Rothenberger D, et al. American Cancer Society guidelines for the early detection of cancer: update of early detection guidelines for prostate, colorectal, and endometrial cancers. Also: update 2001-testing for early lung cancer detection [published erratum appears in CA Cancer J Clin 2001;51:150]. CA Cancer J Clin 2001;51:38-75; quiz 77-80.
*See Table 1.   **See box at end

Leading Causes of Morbidity:
- Acne
- Asthma
- Chlamydia
- Diabetes mellitus
- Headache
- Infective, viral, and parasitic diseases
- Mental disorders, including affective and neurotic disorders
- Nose, throat, ear and upper respiratory infections
- Sexual assault
- Sexually transmitted deseases
- Urinary tract infections
- Vaginitis

Please see page 10 for High-Risk Factors

AGES 19-39 YEARS

SCREENING

History
- Reason for visit
- Health status: medical, surgical, family
- Dietary/nutrition assessment
- Physical activity
- Use of complementary and alternative medicine
- Tobacco, alcohol, other drug use
- Abuse/neglect
- Sexual practices
- Urinary and fecal incontinence

Physical Examination
- Height and weight
- Blood pressure
- Neck, adenopathy, thyroid
- Breasts/abdomen
- Pelvic examination
- Skin*

LABORATORY TESTING

Periodic
- Cervical cytology (annually beginning no later than age 21 years; every 2-3 years after 3 consecutive negative test results if age 30 years or older with no history of cervical intraepithelial neoplasia 2 or 3, immunosuppression, human immunodeficiency virus (HIV) infection, or diethylstilbestrol exposure in utero)+

High-Risk Groups *
- Hemoglobin level assessment
- Bacteriuria testing
- Mammography
- Fasting glucose testing
- Cholesterol testing
- Sexually transmitted disease testing
- Human immunodeficiency testing
- Genetic testing/counseling
- Rubella titer assessment
- Tuberculosis skin testing
- Lipid profile assessment
- Thyroid-stimulating hormone screening

- Hepatitis C virus testing
- Colorectal cancer screening
- Bone density screening

EVALUATION AND COUNSELING

Sexuality
- High-risk behaviors
- Contraceptive options for prevention of unwanted pregnancy, including emergency contraception
- Preconceptional and genetic counseling for desired pregnancy
- Sexually transmitted diseases
  - Partner selection
  - Barrier protection
- Sexual function

Fitness and Nutrition
- Dietary/nutritional assessment
- Exercise: discussion of program
- Folic acid supplementation (0.4 mg/d)
- Calcium intake

Psychosocial Evaluation
- Interpersonal/family relationships
- Domestic violence
- Work satisfaction
- Lifestyle/stress
- Sleep disorders

Cardiovascular Risk Factors
- Family history
- Hypertension
- Dyslipidemia or Obesity
- Diabetes mellitus
- Lifestyle

Health/Risk Behaviors
- Hygiene (including dental)
- Injury prevention
  - Safety belts and helmets
  - Occupational hazards
  - Recreational hazards/firearms
  - Hearing
  - Exercise and sports involvement
- Breast self-examination
- Chemoprophylaxis for breast cancer (for high-risk women ages 35 years or older)
- Skin exposure to ultraviolet rays
- Suicide: depressive symptoms
- Tobacco, alcohol, other drug use

IMMUNIZATIONS

Periodic
- Tetanus-diphtheria booster (every 10 years)

High-Risk Groups *
- Measles, mumps, rubella vaccine
- Hepatitis A virus vaccine
- Hepatitis B virus vaccine
- Influenza vaccine
- Pneumococcal or Varicella vaccine

Please see page 10 for High-Risk Factors

MANAGING CONTRACEPTION

Leading Causes of Death:
- Malignant neoplasms
- Accidents
- Diseases of the heart
- Suicide
- Human immunodeficiency virus infection
- Homicide

Leading Causes of Morbidity:
- Acne
- Appendicitis
- Arthritis/Asthma
- Back symptoms
- Cancer/Chlamydia
- Depression
- Diabetes mellitus
- Gynecologic disorders
- Headache/migraines
- Hypertension
- Infective, viral, and parasitic diseases
- Joint disorders
- Menstrual disorders
- Mental disorders, including affective and neurotic disorders
- Nose, throat, ear, and upper respiratory infections
- Obesity
- Sexual assault/domestic violence
- Sexually transmitted diseases
- Skin rash/dermatitis
- Substance abuse
- Urinary tract infections

AGES 40-64 YEARS

SCREENING
History
- Reason for visit
- Health status: medical, surgical, family
- Dietary/nutrition assessment
- Physical activity
- Use of complementary and alternative medicine
- Tobacco, alcohol, other drug use
- Abuse/neglect
- Sexual practices
- Urinary and fecal incontinence

Physical Examination
- Height, Weight, Blood pressure
- Oral cavity, Neck: adenopathy, thyroid
- Breasts, Axillae, Abdomen, Pelvic examination
- Skin*

LABORATORY TESTING
Periodic
- Cervical cytology (every 2-3 years after 3 consecutive negative test results if no history of cervical intraepithelial neoplasia 2 or 3, immunosuppression, human immunodeficiency virus (HIV) infection, or diethylstilbestrol exposure in utero)+
- Mammography (every 1-2 years beginning at age 40 years; yearly beginning at age 50 years)
- Lipid profile assessment (every 5 years beginning at age 45 years)
- Yearly fecal occult blood testing or flexible sigmoidoscopy every 5 years or yearly fecal occult blood testing plus flexible sigmoidoscopy every 5 years or double contrast barium enema every 5 years or colonoscopy every 10 years (beginning at age 50 years)
- Fasting glucose testing (every 3 years after age 45)
- Thyroid-stimulating hormone screening (every 5 years beginning at age 50 years)

High-Risk Groups *
- Hemoglobin level assessment
- Bacteriuria testing
- Fasting glucose testing
- Sexually transmitted disease testing
- Bone density screening
- HIV/TB testing
- Lipid profile assessment
- Thyroid-stimulating hormone screening
- Hepatitis C virus testing
- Colorectal cancer screening

EVALUATION AND COUNSELING
Sexuality+
- High-risk behaviors
- Contraceptive options for prevention of unwanted pregnancy, including emergency contraception
- Sexually transmitted diseases
    - Partner selection
    - Barrier protection
- Sexual functioning

Fitness and Nutrition
- Dietary/nutrition assessment
- Exercise: discussion of program
- Folic acid supplementation (0.4 mg/d until age 50 years), Calcium intake

Psychosocial Evaluation
- Family relationships, Domestic violence
- Work satisfaction, Retirement planning
- Lifestyle/stress, Sleep disorders

Cardiovascular Risk Factors
- Family history
- Hypertension
- Dyslipidemia or Obesity
- Diabetes mellitus
- Lifestyle

Health/Risk Behaviors
- Hygiene (including dental)
- Hormone therapy
- Injury prevention
    - Safety belts and helmets
    - Occupational hazards
    - Exercise and sports involvement
    - Firearms
    - Hearing

+Preconception counseling is appropriate for certain women in this age group.

* Please see page 10 for High Risk Factors.

7

- Breast self-examination[+++]
- Chemoprophylaxis for breast cancer (for high risk women)
- Skin exposure to ultraviolet rays
- Suicide: depressive symptoms
- Tobacco, alcohol, other drug use

IMMUNIZATIONS
Periodic
- Influenza vaccine (annually beginning at age 50)
- Tetanus-diphtheria booster (every 10 yrs)

High-Risk Groups *
- Measles, mumps, rubella vaccine
- Hepatitis A virus vaccine, Hepatitis B virus vaccine
- Influenza vaccine, Pneumococcal vaccine
- Varicella vaccine

Leading Causes of Death:
- Malignant neoplasms
- Diseases of the heart
- Cerebrovascular diseases
- Chronic lower respiratory disease
- Diabetes mellitus
- Accidents
- Chronic liver disease and cirrhosis
- Suicide
- Human immunodeficiency virus (HIV) disease

Leading Causes of Morbidity:
- Arthritis/osteoarthritis
- Asthma
- Back symptoms
- Cancer
- Cardiovascular disease
- Depression
- Diabetes mellitus
- Headache/migraine
- Hypertension
- Menopause
- Mental disorders, including affective and neurotic disorders
- Mononeuritis of upper limb and mononeuritis multiplex
- Nose, throat, and upper respiratory infections
- Obesity
- Pneumonia
- Sexually transmitted diseases
- Skin conditions/dermatitis
- Ulcers
- Urinary tract infections
- Vision impairment

AGE 65 YEARS AND OLDER

SCREENING
History
- Reason for visit
- Health status: medical, surgical, family
- Dietary/nutritional assessment
- Physical activity
- Use of complementary and alternative medicine
- Tobacco, alcohol, other drug use, and concurrent medication use
- Abuse/neglect
- Sexual practices
- Urinary and fecal incontinence

Physical Examination
- Height, Weight, Blood pressure
- Oral cavity,
- Neck: adenopathy, thyroid
- Breasts, axillae
- Abdomen
- Pelvic examination
- Skin*

LABORATORY TESTING
Periodic
- Cervical cytology (every 2-3 years after 3 consecutive negative test results if no history of cervical intraepithelial neoplasia 2 or 3, immuno-suppression, human immunodeficiency virus (HIV) infection, or diethylstilbestrol exposure in utero)[+]
- Urinalysis
- Mammography
- Lipid profile assessment (every 5 years)
- Yearly fecal occult blood testing or flexible sigmoidoscopy every 5 years or yearly fecal occult blood testing plus flexible sigmoidoscopy every 5 years or double contrast barium enema every 5 years or colonoscopy every 10 years
- Fasting glucose testing (every 3 years)
- Bone density screening
- Thyroid-stimulating hormone screening (every 5 years)

High-Risk Groups *
- Hemoglobin level assessment
- Sexually transmitted disease testing
- Human immunodeficiency virus testing
- Tuberculosis skin testing
- Thyroid-stimulating hormone testing
- Hepatitis C virus testing
- Colorectal cancer screening

* Please see page 10 for High Risk Factors

[+++] Despite a lack of definitive data for or against breast self-examination, breast self-examination has the potential to detect palpable breast cancer and can be recommended.

EVALUATION AND COUNSELING

Sexuality
- Sexual functioning
- Sexual behaviors
- Sexually transmitted diseases
  Partner selection
  Barrier protection

Fitness and Nutrition
- Dietary/nutrition assessment
- Exercise: discussion of program
- Calcium intake

Psychosocial Evaluation
- Neglect/abuse
- Lifestyle/stress
- Depression/sleep disorders
- Family relationships
- Work/retirement satisfaction

Cardiovascular Risk Factors
- Hypertension
- Dyslipidemia or Obesity
- Diabetes mellitus
- Sedentary lifestyle

Health/Risk Behaviors
- Hygiene (including dental)
- Hormone therapy
- Injury prevention
  Safety belts and helmets
  Prevention of falls
  Occupational & Recreational hazards
  Exercise and sports involvement
  Firearms
- Visual acuity/glaucoma; Hearing
- Breast self-examination
- Chemoprophylaxis for breast cancer (for high risk women)
- Skin exposure to ultraviolet rays
- Suicide: depressive symptoms
- Tobacco, alcohol, other drug use

IMMUNIZATIONS

Periodic
- Tetanus-diphtheria booster (every 10 yrs)
- Influenza vaccine (annually)
- Pneumococcal vaccine (once)

High-Risk Groups *
- Hepatitis A virus vaccine
- Hepatitis B virus vaccine
- Varicella vaccine

Leading Causes of Death:
- Diseases of the heart
- Malignant neoplasms
- Cerebrovascular diseases
- Chronic lower respiratory diseases
- Alzheimer's disease
- Influenza and pneumonia
- Diabetes mellitus
- Accidents and adverse effects
- Alzheimer's disease

Leading Causes of Morbidity:
- Arthritis/osteoarthritis
- Asthma
- Back symptoms
- Cancer
- Cardiovascular disease
- Chronic obstructive pulmonary diseases
- Diabetes mellitus
- Hearing and vision impairment
- Hypertension
- Mental disorders, including affective and neurotic disorders
- Nose, throat, and upper respiratory infections
- Obesity/Osteoporosis
- Pneumonia/Septicemia
- Skin lesion/dermatoses/dermatitis
- Ulcers
- Urinary tract infections
- Urinary tract (other conditions, including urinary incontinence)
- Vertigo

* Please see page 10 for High Risk Factors

Sources of Leading Causes of Mortality & Morbidity

Leading causes of mortality are provided by teh Mortality Statistics Branch at the National Center for Health Statistics. Data are from 2000, the most recent year for which final data are available. The causes are ranked.

Leading causes of morbidity are unranked estimates based on information fromt he following sources:
- National Health Interview Survey, 1998
- National Ambulatory Medical Care Survey, 2001
- National Health and Nutrition Examination Survey III, 1998
- National Hospital Discharge Survey, 2001
- National Nursing Home Survey, 1997
- U.S. Department of Justice National Crime Victimization Survey
- U.S. Centers for Disease Control and Prevention Sexually Transmitted Disease Surveillance, 2001
- U.S. Centers for Disease Control and Prevention HIV/AIDS Surveillance Report, 2001

INTERVENTIONS FOR HIGH-RISK FACTORS

Intervention	High-Risk Factor
• Bacteriuria testing	Diabetes mellitus
• Bone density screening	Postmenopausal women younger than 65 years: personal history of fracture as an adult; history of fracture in a first-degree relative; Caucasian; dementia; poor health or frailty; current cigarette smoking; low body weight (<127 lb); estrogen deficiency caused by early (age <45 years) menopause, bilateral ovariectomy, or prolonged (>1 year) premenopausal amenorrhea; low life-long calcium intake; alcoholism; impaired eyesight despite adequate correction; recurrent falls; inadequate physical activity. All women: certain diseases or medical conditions and those who take certain drugs associated with an increased risk of osteoporosis
• Colorectal cancer screening	Colorectal cancer or adenomatous polyps in first-degree relative younger than 60 years or in two or more first-degree relatives of any ages; family history of familial adenomatous polyposis or hereditary nonpolyposis colon cancer; history of colorectal cancer, adenomatous polyps, or inflammatory bowel disease, chronic ulcerative colitis, or Crohn's disease
• Fasting glucose test	Overweight (body mass index ≥ 24 kg/m^2); family history of diabetes mellitus; habitual physical inactivity; high-risk race/ethnicity (eg, African American, Hispanic, Native American, Asian, Pacific Islander); have given birth to a new-born weighing more than 9 lb or history of gestational diabetes mellitus; hypertension; high-density lipoprotein cholesterol level ≤ 35 mg/dL; triglyceride level ≥ 250 mg/dL; history of impaired glucose tolerance or impaired fasting glucose; polycystic ovary syndrome; history of vascular disease
• Fluoride supplementation	Live in area with inadequate water fluoridation (<0.7 ppm)
• Genetic testing/counseling	Considering pregnancy and: will be 35 years or older at time of delivery; patient, partner, or family member with history of genetic disorder or birth defect; exposure to teratogens; or African, Acadian, European Caucasian, Eastern European (Ashkenazi) Jewish, Mediterranean, or Southeast Asian ancestry
• Hemoglobin level assessment	Caribbean, Latin American, Asian, Mediterranean, or African ancestry; history of excessive menstrual flow
• Hepatitis A vaccination	Chronic liver disease; clotting factor disorders; illegal drug users; individuals who work with HAV infected nonhuman primates or with HAV in a research laboratory setting; individuals traveling to or working in countries that have high or intermediate endemicity of hepatitis A
• Hepatitis B vaccination	Hemodialysis patients; patients who receive clotting factor concentrates; health care workers and public safety workers who have exposure to blood in the workplace; individuals in training in schools of medicine, dentistry, nursing, laboratory technology, and other allied health professions; injecting drug users; individuals with more than 1 sexual partner in the previous 6 months; individuals with a recently acquired STD; all clients in STD clinics; household contacts and sexual partners of individuals with chronic HBV infection; clients and staff of institutions for the developmentally diabled; international travelers who will be in countries with high or intermediate prevalence or chronic HBV infection for more than 6 months; inmates of correctional facilities
• Hepatitis C virus (HCV) testing	History of injecting illegal drugs; recipients of clotting factor concentrates before 1987; chronic (long-term) hemodialysis; persistently abnormal alanine aminotransferase levels; recipient of blood from a donor who later tested positive for HCV infection; recipient of blood or blood-component transfusion or organ transplant before July 1992; occupational percutaneous or mucosal exposure to HCV-positive blood
• Human immunodeficiency virus (HIV) testing	Seeking treatment for STIs; drug use by injection; history of prostitution; past or present sexual partner who is HIV positive or bisexual or injects drugs; long-term residence or birth in an area with high prevalence of HIV infection; history of transfusion from 1978-1985; invasive cervical cancer. Offer to women seeking preconceptional evaluation

• Influenza vaccination	Anyone who wishes to reduce the chance of becoming ill with influenza; chronic cardiovascular or pulmonary diorders including asthma; chronic metabolic diseases, including diabetes mellitus, renal dysfunction, hemo-globinopathies, and immunosuppression (including immunosupression caused by medications or by HIV); residents of nursing homes and other long-term care facilities; individuals likely to transmit influenza to high risk individuals (eg, household members and caregivers of elderly, those with medical indications, and adults with high-risk conditions); health-care workers; day-care workers
• Lipid profile assessment	Family history suggestive of familial hyperlipidemia; family history of premature (age <50 years for men, <60 years for women) cardiovascular disease; diabetes mellitus; multiple coronary heart disease risk factors (eg, tobacco use, hypertension)
• Mammography	Women who have had breast cancer or who have a first-degree relative (ie, mother, sister, or daughter) or multiple other relatives who have a history of premenopausal breast or breast and ovarian cancer
• Measles, mumps, rubella vaccine	Adults born in 1957 or later should be offered vaccination (one dose of MMR) if there is no proof or immunity or documentation of a dose given after first birthday; persons vaccinated in 1963-1967 should be offered revaccination (2 doses); health-care workers, students entering college, international travelers, and rubella-negative postpartum patients should be offered a second dose
• Pneumococcal vaccine	Chronic illness such as cardiovascular disease, pulmonary disease, diabetes mellitus, alcoholism, chronic liver disease, cerebrospinal fluid leaks, functional asplenia (eg, sickle cell disease) or splenectomy; exposure to an environment where pneumococcal outbreaks have occurred; immuno-compromised patients (eg, HIV infection, hematologic or solid malignancies, chemotherapy, steroid therapy); Revaccination after 5 years may be appropriate for certain high-risk groups
• Rubella titer assessment	Childbearing age and no evidence of immunity
• STD testing	History of multiple sexual partners or a sexual partner with multiple contacts, sexual contact with persons with culture-positive STI, history of repeated episodes of STIs, attendance at clinics for STIs; routine screening for chlamydial infection for all sexually active women aged 25 years or younger and other asymptomatic women at high risk for infection; routine screening for gonorrheal infection for all sexually active adolescents and other asymptomatic women at high risk for infection
• Skin examination	Increased recreational or occupational exposure to sunlight; family or personal history of skin cancer; clinical evidence of precursor lesions
• Thyroid-stimulating hormone test	Strong family history of thyroid disease; autoimmune disease (evidence of subclinical hypothyroidism may be related to unfavorable lipid profiles)
• Tuberculosis skin test	HIV infection; close contact with persons known or suspected to have TB; medical risk factors known to increase risk of disease if infected; born in country with high TB prevalence; medically underserved; low income; alcoholism; intravenous drug use; resident of long-term care facility (e.g., correctional institutions, mental institutions, nursing homes and facilities); health professional working in high-risk health-care facilities
• Varicella vaccine	All susceptible adults and adolescents, including health-care workers; household contacts of immunocompromised individuals; teachers; day-care workers; residents and staff of institutional settings, colleges, prisons, or military installations; adolescents and adults living in households with children; international travellers; non-pregnant women of childbearing age

*For a more detailed discussion of bone density screening, see Bone density screening for osteoporosis. ACOG Committee Opinion No. 270. American College of Obstetricians and Gynecologists. Obstet Gynecol 2002;99:523-5.

**For a more detailed discussion of colorectal cancer screening, see Smith RA, von Eschenbach AC, Wender R, Levin B, Byers T, Rothenberg D, et al. American Cancer Society guidelines for the early detection of cancer: update of early detection guidelines for prostate, colorectal, and endometrial cancers. Also: update 2001-testing for early lung cancer detection [published erratum appears in CA Cancer J Clin 2001;51:150]. CA Cancer J Clin 2001;51:38-75; quiz 77-80.

Advantages of counseling:
- Involves patient in his/her own care and dispels misconceptions, myths and rumors
- Improves success with complicated regimens
- Helps people change risky behaviors— a vital, yet difficult, task
- Facilitates the decision-making process regarding contraception and STI prevention
- Explains possible side effects, which reduces anxiety, increases success with method and encourages clients to return if problems occur, reducing severity of complications
- Builds and strengthens the provider/patient relationship
- Encourages patient responsibility for his/her health decisions
- Ensures and maintains *confidentiality*

Principles of good counseling: Allow plenty of time: important and difficult
- *Listen*, look at your patients, allow them to speak freely, paraphrase what you hear
- Remember LISTEN and SILENT use the same letters!
- *Respect*, recognize and accept each individual's unique situation
- Accept and anticipate that behavior change occurs slowly and incrementally. Remember that *"a lapse is not a relapse;* [Prochaska-1994]
- Remain *sensitive*; acknowledge that sex/sexuality are very personal
- Be *nonjudgmental* and encourage *self-determination;* avoid *false reassurance*
- *Urge all your patients to know their HIV status;* each encounter offers opportunity to counsel about STI/HIV prevention and contraception
- Inquire about problems patients may have had with previous medical recommendations
- Know what you are talking about!
- Realize that your patient will remember only 1-4 points from each visit. Avoid information overload and provide written information at appropriate reading level for later reference

The GATHER method suggests the following steps:
- **Greet** patient in a warm, friendly manner; help her or him to feel at ease
- **Ask** patient about her or his needs and reproductive goals; ask about risk for STIs
- **Tell** patient about her or his choices, explaining the advantages and disadvantages of all options
- **Help** patient to choose
- **Explain** the correct use of the method or drug being prescribed
- **Repeat** important instructions to the patient and clarify time and conditions of return visit; give written instructions to patient to review later

Reproductive/Contraceptive Goals:

GOAL:	MAIN CONTRACEPTIVE CONCERNS MAY BE:
Delaying birth of first child	Effectiveness of method, future fertility and STIs; explain EC
Avoiding abortion	Need for maximal effectiveness; Tell about ECs; May want to use 2 methods consistently
Spacing births	Balance of efficacy and convenience; explain EC
Completed childbearing	Needs effective method for long term

HOW TO PICK A BOYFRIEND:
(The same concept applies, of course, to picking a girlfriend)

Don't even think about it! If he...
- Is a needle user, even once ←
- Uses drugs or gives you drugs
- Is violent
- Committed a serious crime

Don't even talk, don't find out his name, just walk away!

You deserve better! Beware if he...

- Has lots of former girlfriends he had sex with
- Doesn't listen to you
- Doesn't want you to have other friends ←
- Has children that he is not supporting
- Is currently having sex with another person
- Lies to you
- Uses or wants your money or is heavily in debt
- Is extremely disrespectful in referring to his mother
- Refuses to wear a condom
- Lies, blames, is very bossy ←

This could work! If...

- He respects you
- He has a life plan that fits your life plan
- He listens to you
- He never, ever scares you
- He appeals to you

Felicia Guest is a remarkable individual and an extremely creative health educator! Above is an adaptation of her thoughts on how a girl or woman could decide if a boy or man were a bad or good prospect as a date (with credits to Dr. Felicia Stewart): Sometimes, after hearing the above, a teenager will reply, "but I love him." Felicia Guest suggests the following response to the "but I love him" feeling: "Love is NOT supposed to hurt."

If you have shared the above outline with your own or other children, patients or classes, please email your and their response to us at www.managingcontraception.com. Also send us any additions or deletions you might have to HOW TO PICK A BOYFRIEND. Thanks and have ← fun with this teaching tool.

STRUCTURED COUNSELING

Carefully planned structured counseling is very different than counseling.
Structured counseling may involve techniques such as:
- Repetition of a specific message at the time of the initial visit
- Having the patient repeat back her understanding of a message
- Use of a brief, clear, concise videotape
- Asking the patient if she has questions about the videotape
- Written instructions that clearly highlight key messages
- Repetition at each follow-up visit
- Checklist for patient to fill out at *each* follow up visit

Continuation rates among women started on Depo-Provera are low (only
40-60% at one year).*
Methodical structured counseling for women starting on Depo-Provera might include:
- **The message: Depo-Provera will change your periods.** No woman's periods stay the same as they were before starting Depo-Provera. Ask: *"Will you find it acceptable if there are major changes in your periods?"* If no, steer clear of DMPA, continuous COCs, mini pills
- Having the patient repeat back her understanding of parts of one's message, particularly the message that **over time women stop having periods most months**. Women tend to have very irregular menses almost immediately
- Use of a brief, clear, concise videotape
- Asking the patient if she has questions about the videotape
- Written instructions that clearly highlight the key messages
- Asking at each 3-month visit what has happened to a woman's pattern of bleeding, whether amenorrhea has begun and how she feels about her pattern of bleeding

Checklist for Depo-Provera patient to fill out at each follow up visit. Please check yes or no. Tell us if you have:

Spotting or irregular vaginal bleeding	☐ Yes	☐ No
Missed periods or very, very light periods	☐ Yes	☐ No
Concern over your pattern of vaginal bleeding	☐ Yes	☐ No
Depression, severe anxiety or mood changes	☐ Yes	☐ No
Gained 5 pounds or more	☐ Yes	☐ No
Questions you want to ask us about Depo-Provera injections	☐ Yes	☐ No
Have you ever had a wrist, hip or other fracture	☐ Yes	☐ No

* Structured counseling is also important for women starting COCs, patch, NuvaRings, LNG IUD or condoms

See **STRUCTURED COUNSELING** on p. 133 for an analysis of the effect of structured counseling on Depo-Provera discontinuation rates

CHAPTER 4

Taking Sexual Histories

More clinicians are realizing that sexual histories are essential to identifying at-risk individuals and to providing appropriate testing and treatment. Explain to the patient that obtaining sexual information is necessary to provide complete care, but reassure her or him that she or he has the right to discuss only what she/he is comfortable divulging. Ask patients less direct questions in the beginning to build trust, then ask the questions that explicitly address sexual issues once you have their confidence. Be cautious about what **information** you place on the chart. Medical records are not necessarily confidential and can be reviewed by insurance companies **(may also be subpoenaed in legal proceedings)**

Initiating the Sexual History

- I will be asking some personal questions about your sexual activity to help me make more accurate diagnoses. This is a normal part of the exam I do with all patients
- To help keep accurate medical records, I will be writing down some of your responses. If there are things you do not want me to record, you only need to tell me as much as you are comfortable sharing
- Some patients have shared concerns with me related to their risks of infections or concerns about particular sexual activities. If you have any concerns, I would be happy to discuss them with you

Sexual History Questions

- **What are you doing to protect yourself from HIV and other infections? OR**
  What are you doing to put yourself at risk for AIDS?
- Do you have questions regarding sex or sexual activity?
- How old were you when you had your first sexual experience?
- Do you have sex with men, women or both?
- Do you need contraception? How are you protecting yourself from unwanted pregnancy?
- How many sex partners have you had in the last 3 months? in the last 6 months? in your lifetime?
- How many sex partners does your partner have?
- Do you have penis in vagina sex? penis in mouth sex? or penis in rectum sex?
- Do you drink alcohol or take drugs in association with sexual activity?
- Have you ever been forced or coerced to have sex?
- Are you now in a relationship where you feel physically, sexually, or emotionally threatened or abused?
- When you were younger, did anyone touch your private body parts or ask you to touch theirs?
- Have you ever had sex for money, food, protection, drugs or shelter?
- Do you enjoy sex? Do you usually have orgasms? Do you ever have pain with sex?
- Do you or your partner(s) have any sexual concerns?

Avoid Assumptions: Making assumptions about a patient's sexual behavior and orientation can leave out important information, undermine patient trust and make the patient feel judged or alienated, causing her to withhold information. This can result in diagnostic and treatment errors. Do not assume that patients:

- ARE sexually active and need contraception
- Are NOT sexually active (e.g., older patients, young adolescents)
- Are heterosexual, homosexual or bisexual OR know if their partners have other partners
- Have power (within a relationship) to make or implement their own contraceptive decisions

FEMALE

Dyspareunia

- *Definition:* Pain during vaginal intercourse or vaginal penetration
- *Key questions:* Does she have pain with vaginal penetration? Does she have pain with early entry or in the mid vaginal area? Is there pain with deep thrusting? Is pain occasional or consistent? With every partner? Does the pain change with different sexual positions? Is she aroused and lubricated before penetration?
- *Causes:* Organic - vestibulitis, urethritis/UTI, vaginitis, cervicitis, vulvodynia, interstitial cystitis, traumatic deliveries (forcep or vacuum extractions), hypoestrogenism, PID, endometriosis, surgical scars or adhesions, pelvic injuries, tumors, hip joint or disc pain, female circumcision, orgasmic spasm, lack of foreplay, lubrication
Psychological - current or previous abuse, relationship stress, depression, anxiety, fear of sex or fear of pregnancy
- *Treatment:* Directed to underlying pathology including depression. If dyspareunia is chronic, consider supplementing medical management with supportive counseling and sex therapy

Vaginismus (special case of dyspareunia)

- *Definition:* Painful involuntary spastic contraction of introital and pelvic floor muscles
- *Causes:* Organic - may be secondary to current or previous dyspareunia and its causes. Psychological - sexual abuse, fears of abnormal anatomy (e.g. terror that vagina will rip with penile or speculum introduction), negative attitudes about sexuality
- *Treatment:* Education is critical. Insight into underlying causes helps. After source is recognized, start progressive desensitization exercises, which can include self manipulation and dilators. Sex therapist/psychologist intervention may be needed to deal with unconscious fears unresponsive to education

Decreased Libido (Hypoactive Sexual Desire)

- *Definition:* Relative lack of sexual desire defined by individual as troublesome to her sexual relationship; there is no absolute "normal" level
- *Causes:* **Organic** - may be due to acute or chronic debilitating medical condition (e.g., diabetes, stroke, spinal cord injury, arthritis, pain, cancer, chronic obstructive pulmonary disease, coronary artery disease, etc.), medications (e.g. sedatives, narcotics, hypnotics, anticonvulsants, centrally-acting antihypertensives, tranquilizers, anorectics, oral contraceptives, Depo-Provera, and some antidepressants), dyspareunia, incontinence, alcohol, hormonal imbalance, or healing episiotomy or other surgical scars; Sexual practices - inadequate sexualstimulation or time for arousal. Sexual desires discordant with partner's desires
Psychological - depression, anxiety, exhaustion, life stress (finances, relationship problems, etc.), poor partner communications, lack of understanding about impacts of aging. Change in body image (breast-feeding, postpartum, weight gain, cancer, or post mastectomy or hysterectomy)
- *Treatment:* Treat underlying causes where possible. Rule out hyperactive sexual desire disorder of partner. Reassure about normalcy, if appropriate. Help patient create time and special space for sexual expression - no distractions from children, telephone, household chores. Suggest variety in sexual practices perhaps with aid of fantasies (romantic novels, films, etc). Physiologic androgen replacement has never been found in a controlled trial to enhance libido in oophrectomized women. New drugs and creams, causing increased blood flow to the clitoris, may increase sexual arousal for those women whose problems started after developing a medical disorder and had normal function previously. Consider

referral to sex therapist. Read *For Each Other* by Lonnie Barbach and *Women, Sex & Desire* by Elizabeth Davis or *Our Bodies, Ourselves*

Excessive Sexual Desire (Hyperactive Sexual Desire)
- *Definition:* Excessive sexual activity resulting in social, psychological and physical problems. See Diagnostic and Statistical Manual of Mental Disorders, Fourth Edition (DSM-IV)
- *Cause:* Low self esteem; abuse; attention seeking; acting out; mania; bipolar disease
- *Treatment:* Refer for psychological counseling and therapy, Sex Addicts Anonymous after therapy

Orgasmic Disorders: Anorgasmia or Primary Anorgasmia
- *Definitions:*
  - *Preorgasmia or Primary Anorgasmia:* Never experienced orgasms and desires to be orgasmic
  - *Secondary Anorgasmia:* Orgasmic in past, no orgasms currently, desirous of orgasm
- *Cause:* Organic - may be secondary to dyspareunia, neurological, vascular disease, medications (e.g. sedatives, narcotics, hypnotics, anticonvulsants, centrally-acting antihypertensives, tranquilizers, anorectics, and some antidepressants - particularly SSRI class antidepressants), or poor sexual techniques of partner (painful, rapid ejaculation) Psychological - negative attitude about sexuality, chronic relationship stress; lack of knowledge about body and sexual response
- *Treatment:* Treat underlying organic causes, if possible. Explain sexual response (suggest reading *Our Bodies, Ourselves*). Add behavioral/psychological approach using PLISSIT model (see Abbreviations, p. x), and sensate focusing exercises. Help couple set alternative pleasuring goals. Refer to sex therapist if initial interventions not successful. Have woman learn how to have an orgasm on her own in comfortable environment and then she can teach her partner how to pleasure her. Recommend use of lubricants, vibrators and sex toys. Read *For Yourself* by Lonnie Barbach

MALE
Decreased Libido (Hypoactive sexual desire disorder)
- No absolute level is "normal"; "decreased libido" is usually related to previous experience, partner's expectations, or perceived societal norms
- Evaluation and treatment similar to female's (see above)

Excessive Sexual Desire (Hyperactive Sexual Desire)
- *Definition:* Excessive sexual activity resulting in social, psychological and physical problems.
- *Cause:* Abuse at young age; attention seeking; acting out; mania; other such as bipolar disease
- *Treatment:* Refer for psychological counseling and therapy, Sex Addicts Anonymous after therapy

Premature (Rapid) Ejaculation
- *Definition:* Recurrent ejaculation before or shortly after vaginal penetration or ejaculation occurs earlier than patient or partner desires. Average time from entry to ejaculation in "normal" couples is 2 minutes; shorter interval is consistent with diagnosis.
- *Causes:* Organic - urethritis, prostatitis, neurological disease (e.g. multiple sclerosis). Psychological - learned behavior, result of anxiety (especially among teens)
- *Treatment:* Education and reassurance is important. If goal is pleasuring of partner, teach other techniques to arouse her or him prior to intercourse and/or to achieve orgasm. "Start and stop" technique can be used to prolong erection; man stops stimulation for at least 30 seconds when he feels ejaculation imminent. "Squeeze" technique helpful; when man feels impending ejaculation, partner firmly squeezes the head of the penis beneath the glans for 4-5 seconds to decrease erection. Selective serotonin reuptake inhibitors (SSRIs) in low doses may be helpful if these other techniques are not adequate. Refer to sex therapist (or urologist if cause organic) for additional treatment if needed. Condoms are available with benzocaine to decrease sensation and reduce premature ejaculation

Delayed (Retarded) Ejaculation/Anorgasmia
- *Definition:* Inability to or difficulty in experiencing orgasm and ejaculation with a partner
- *Cause:* usually psychological; learned behavior; may occur when a man has masturbatory patterns that cannot be duplicated with partner; overemphasis on sexual performance; medications such as SSRI's. Rule out organic problems carefully
- *Treatment:* referral to sex therapist recommended

Erectile Dysfunction/Disorders (ED) (Impotence)
- *Definition:* Inability to attain or sustain an erection that is satisfactory for coitus
- *Primary:* never achieved erection
- *Causes:* Organic - low testosterone levels due to hypothalamic-pituitary-testicular disorder; severe vascular compromise. Psychological - usual cause
- *Secondary:* current inability to attain or maintain erection (may be situational)
- *Causes:* Organic - diabetes mellitus, alcohol abuse, hypothyroidism, drug dependency, medications (e.g. sedatives, narcotics, hypnotics, anticonvulsants, centrally-acting antihypertensives, tranquilizers, anorectics, and some antidepressants), hypopituitarism, penile infections, atherosclerosis, aortic aneurysm, multiple sclerosis, spinal cord lesions, orchiectomy or prostatectomy
  Psychological - depression, relationship stress, prior abuse, etc. Suspect when patient has morning erection or is able to masturbate to ejaculation
- *Treatment:* Treat underlying cause. Switch medications if possible. Same measures that help women's sexual desire may be useful. Medical or mechanical treatments available:
  1. *Testosterone.* Shown to be useful in wasting diseases (AIDS) and other low testosterone conditions. Available in patches for ease of use
  2. *Phosphodiesterase inhibitors:* Viagra, Cialis, Levitra ◄──
  3. *Alprostadil injections (Edex or Caverject)* prostaglandin E1 ~ 1 cc injected into corpus cavernosa (strengths 125 µg - 1000 µg). Excessive injection may cause priapism. Erection achieved with stimulation lasts 30-60 minutes. Avoid in anticoagulated patients and with vasoactive medications.
  4. *Alprostadil suppository (Muse)* prostaglandin pellet E1 (125-1000 µg) placed inside urethra. Erection occurs as drug absorbed. 70% successful. Contraindications - anatomical penile abnormalities (strictures, hypospadias, etc.), and thrombosis risk factors. Limit 2/day
  5. *Yohimbine hydrochloride.* Prescription pill composed of indole alkaloid. Modestly successful. Avoid in psychiatric patients.
  6. *Vacuum Erection Device (VED).* Use of a vacuum pump and different size rubber bands maintains an erection for 30 minutes. Safe and effective (90% success rate).
  7. *Penile implants (prostheses).* Permanent bendable rods or inflatable reservoirs implanted surgically into penis. Activated/inflated for intercourse. Success rate high, but associated with surgical risks and the risk that natural erections disappear
  8. *Microsurgery.* Used in men with atherosclerosis of penile arteries or venous pathology; over 50% success rate

CHAPTER 6
Adolescent Issues
advocatesforyouth.org, youngwomenshealth.org, teenwire.com,
arhp.org/arhpframepated.htm, www.askdurex.com

Adolescents are very interested in sex, contraception, and STIs, but they rarely raise these issues with their providers. Abstinence (delaying first intercourse) is increasing slightly among male and female teens, but most American adolescents have had intercourse before high school graduation. Helping adolescents to grow in self respect, is the most important goal of all who work with teens.

COUNSELING CHALLENGES POSED BY ADOLESCENTS

Teens are not "young adults." Developmentally appropriate approaches are needed
- Age 12-14 – teens are very concrete, egocentric (self-focused) and concerned with personal appearance and acceptance, and have a short attention span
- Age 14-15 – teens are peer oriented and authority resistant (challenge boundaries), and have very limited images of the future
- Age 16-17 – teens are developing logical thought processes and goals for the future

Nonjudgmental, open-ended and reflective questions are better than direct yes-no inquiries. Try reflective questions such as "What would you want to tell a friend who was thinking about having sex?" instead of "You're not having sex, are you?"

CONFIDENTIALITY:
Adolescents are often afraid to obtain medical care for contraception, pregnancy testing or STI treatment because they fear parental reaction. Over two-thirds of teens never discuss with their parents anything sexual that they have done; over one-half feel that their parents could not handle it. All teens should be entitled to confidential services and counseling, but billing systems and/or laws in some states affect their confidential access to family planning services. Know your local laws and refer to sites that may be able to meet all the teen's needs if your practice can not.

ADOLESCENTS AND THE LAW:
This table provides information on an adolescent's right to consent to reproductive health, contraception, and abortion services.

Table 6.1 Adolescents and the Law

AL ●■□★	DC ●■+	IA ○■+	MI ○■□★	NH ●■◇	OK ●■□◇	TX ○■□+
AK ●■★	FL ●■◇	KS ●■□+	MN ●■◇	NJ ●□◇	OR ●■+	UT ○■+
AZ ●■★	GA ●■□+	KY ●■★	MS ●■★	NM ○■◇	PA ●■★	VT ○■+
AR ●■□+	HI ●■+	LA ○■●★	MO ●□●	NY ●■+	RI ○■★	VA ●■+
CA ●■+	ID ○■★	ME ●■□+	MT ●■◇	NC ○■★	SC ●■★	WA ●■+
CO ●■+	IL ●■◇	MD ●■★	NE ○■★	ND ○■★	SD ○■+	WV ●■+
CT ◇■+	IN ○■★	MA ●■★	NV ●■◇	OH ○■□+	TN ●■★	WI ○■★
DE ●■+						WY ●■★

● = Minor may consent to contraceptive service (including some states with special circumstances such as the minors' age, health, marital, or pregnancy status)
○ = No explicit policy related to minors' access to contraceptive services
■ = Minor may consent to testing and treatment for STDs
□ = Physician may inform parents about STD testing and treatment but is not required to
★ = Parental consent required before a minor may obtain an abortion
☆ = Parental consent law exists but not in effect (e.g., declared unenforceable by courts)
+ = Parental notification required before a minor may obtain an abortion. In some states, parental notification is not necessary if a risk for the minor is perceived (i.e. telling parents may result in harm to minor)
◇ = Parental notification law exists but not in effect (e.g., declared unenforceable by courts)
+ = Does not require parental involvement before a minor may obtain an abortion

Sources: State Policies in Brief: Parental Involvement in Minors' Abortions; Minors' Access to STD Services; Minors' Access to Contraceptive Services. As of February 1, 2004. Alan Guttmacher Institute.

Note: Many of the laws contain specific clauses that affect their meaning and application. The authors encourage readers to consult the above documents (updated monthly) for more details: www.agi-usa.org.

PELVIC EXAMS AND BIRTH CONTROL PILLS

The pelvic exam may be a barrier to initiating contraceptive use. It is not necessary to perform a pelvic exam prior to prescribing pills [Stewart-2001]

ADOLESCENTS AS RISK TAKERS

- Full evaluation of behaviors is important to personalize counseling. Teens must move away from parental authority figures to become independent adult individuals, but, along the way, they may take excessive risks in many areas, including sexuality
- HEADSS interview technique helpful as an organized approach. Ask each teen about Home, Education, Activities, Drugs, Sexuality (activity, orientation and abuse) and Suicide
- Look for the female athletic triad: eating disorders, amenorrhea and osteoporosis. This triad of symptoms may also occur in women who do not exercise excessively
- Provide emergency contraceptive pills in advance ←

SEX EDUCATION

Sex education has been abbreviated in most U.S. schools, sometimes focusing entirely on an "abstinence-only" message. Moreover, sex education, contraception and STIs curricula offered in many schools sometimes are not medically correct. The information teens obtain from peers is also often inaccurate. Common **MYTHS** are:

- *You cannot get pregnant the first time you have intercourse*
- *You cannot get pregnant if you douche after sex*
- *Having a baby makes you a woman, makes your boyfriend love you, and gets you the attention you deserve*
- *Making a girl pregnant means that you are a man*

Adolescents need very concrete information and opportunities to role play and practice:

- How to open and place a condom and where to carry it
- How to negotiate NOT having sex and, in other cases, condom use
- How to punch out the pills, where to keep the pack, and how to remember them
- The remarkable advantages of extended use of pills, and the disadvantages of this approach as well
- How to move in direction of dual protection: condoms and another contraceptive
- How to use emergency contraception, the patch and the vaginal ring

TEEN BIRTH RATES AND ABORTION RATES ←

U.S. teens experience first sexual intercourse at about the same time and have more partners than teens in many other developed countries. However, teen birth, teen abortion, and sexually transmitted infection (STI) rates in the United States are higher than in most other industrialized countries. In 1999, 48 out of 1000 U.S. women ages 15-19 gave birth— a rate 11 times greater than in the Netherlands and four times higher than in Germany. The teen abortion rate in the U.S. is more than three times that of France and nearly seven times that of the Netherlands. [Advocates for Youth-2005]

Nation	Teen Birth Rates (1999) (per 1000 women ages 15-19)	Teen Abortion Rates (per 1000 women ages 15-19) ←
United States	48.7	27.5
Netherlands	4.5	4.2
Germany	12.5	3.6
France	10.0	10.2

CHAPTER 7
Male Reproductive Health ←

Reproductive health is a term generally associated with women. Recently, efforts have been made to include males in health education and outreach programs, acknowledging that men have important reproductive and sexual health needs of their own. Including men in discussions of contraception and STIs benefits their female partners as well.

MEN AND SEXUAL EXPERIENCE ←

• Most adult men and half of adolescent men have had sexual intercourse.
• For men in the United States: Average first intercourse – 16.9 years old
  Average first marriage – 26.7 years old
• So…many young men are sexually active for 10 years before marriage.
• Almost one quarter of male adolescents initiate sex by age 15. *(Sonfield, 2002)*

WHERE MEN GET THEIR REPRODUCTIVE HEALTH INFORMATION ←

• Of 15-19 year old males, 71% had physical exams in the past year but only 39% received reproductive health services. *(Porter, 2000)*
• One-third of men aged 18-44 have no regular doctor, another one-third have not seen a physician in the past year. *(Sonfield, 2002)*
• Men are less likely than women to have health insurance. *(Sonfield, 2002)*
• One survey showed men get most of their STD/AIDS prevention information from the media rather than from a healthcare provider. *(Bradner, 2000)*
• Although most men get some form of sexuality education while they are in high school, for 3 out of 10 men this instruction comes too late – after they have begun having sexual intercourse. *(Sonfield, 2002)*

What can healthcare providers do?
• Make sure to talk to men about reproductive health at school and work physicals. ←
  Start early – many adolescents have sexual intercourse before age 17.
• When appropriate, talk to men about reproductive health issues such as STIs and contraception at doctor's visits for unrelated complaints – this may be the only time they visit a physician this year!

MEN AND CONTRACEPTION

• Among sexually experienced adolescent males, 14% have made a partner pregnant and ← 2-7% are fathers. *(Marcell, 2003)*
• 38% of men aged 25-49 report their last child was mistimed or unwanted. *(Sonfield, 2002)*
• As men get older, condom use declines. 7 out of 10 men age 15-17 use condoms, compared to 4 out of 10 men in their 20s, and 2 out of 10 men in their 30s. *(Sonfield, 2002)*
• Vasectomy is a very effective male option for permanent birth control. However, it is estimated that approximately 500,000 men receive a vasectomy in the U.S. each year, in contrast to 700,000 women who have a female sterilization procedure. *(Hawes, 1998)* In only 4 countries throughout the world, Great Britain, Netherlands, New Zealand and Bhutan, do vasectomies exceed tubal sterilization as a method of birth control. Vasectomy has not been found to cause any long-term adverse effects ←

Men's support of women's birth control methods matter

• Education of adolescent males about birth control (including female methods) leads to improvement in use of the method by their partner(s). Adolescent females who always talk to their male partners were at lowest risk of pregnancy and STIs, and those who did not were at highest risk. *(Edwards, 1994)*

MEN AND SEXUALLY TRANSMITTED INFECTIONS

How many men acquire sexually transmitted infections?

• 17% of men aged 15-49 have genital herpes ◀━━
• Among men in their 20s, there are 500-600 new cases of gonorrhea and chlamydia per year, per 100,000 men *(Sonfield, 2002)*
• 8 out of 10 Americans living with HIV are men *(Sonfield, 2002)* ◀━━
• Rates of STIs are higher among young, poor, and minority men

Decreasing STI rates in men helps their female partner(s)

• Treating men decreases initial infection rate and reinfection rate in women, which could decrease female complications such as pelvic inflammatory disease, ectopic pregnancy, and infertility.

Decreasing STI rates in men helps themselves

• While the link between gonorrhea and chlamydia infection and infertility in men has not been proven, there is some clinical evidence that it does have some effect:
  gonorrhea/chlamydia infection ➤ urethritis ➤ epidymo-orchitis ➤ infertility
  • If urethritis is treated promptly, there is less likelihood it will proceed to epidymo-orchitis *(Ness, 1997)*
  • The most common cause of epidymo-orchitis in men younger than 35 years old is gonorrhea and chlamydia infections *(Weidner, 1999)*

MEN AND REPRODUCTIVE CANCERS

Testicular cancer

• "Testicular cancer is the most common solid malignancy affecting males between the ◀━━ ages of 15 and 35, although it accounts for only 1% of all cancers in men." *(Michaelson, 2004)*
• The number of deaths from testicular has dropped recently from advances in therapy. ◀━━
• Some signs or symptoms of testicular cancer are testicular enlargement, a dull ache in the abdomen or groin, scrotal pain, and fluid in the scrotum.
• The patient information website sponsored by the American Urological Association says that monthly testicular self exams are the most important way to detect a tumor early.
• The treatment for testicular cancer can be removal of the affected testicle. Removal of one testicle does not make a man infertile.

Prostate cancer

• The most important risk factor for prostate cancer is age. The older a man is, the greater his risk.
• Prostate cancer is screened for by digital rectal exam and prostate-specific antigen level.
• Some of the treatments for prostate cancer can affect male fertility. For instance, surgery to remove the prostate causes the male ejaculate to become "dry" so the ability to have children is usually lost. Prostate surgery can also cause erectile dysfunction ◀━━

PERIMENOPAUSE: The 3-5 years toward the end of the reproductive life of a woman and the first 12 months after the last menstrual period. An important marker of the perimenopause is menstrual irregularity. The hallmark of this period is fluctuations in ovarian hormones resulting in intermittent vasomotor symptoms, menstrual disturbances and reduced fertility. A perimenopausal woman needs contraception until she is truly menopausal (no menses x 1 yr). Perimenopausal women have the highest abortion rate (# abortions/ # pregnancies) of any group except women under 15

- All methods of birth control are available to healthy nonsmoking women until menopause
- In the United States, 50% of all contracepting women age 40-44 have been sterilized and another 20% have a partner with a vasectomy
- Oral contraceptive pills, patches, rings, hormonal IUDs, or combined injections may provide the additional benefits of control of DUB, prevention of osteoporosis, hot flashes and irregular cycles. Estrogen-containing contraceptives should not be used in women over 35 who smoke or have significant CV risk factors.
- Smokers over 35 may use POPs or DMPA, IUDs, or barriers
- WHO (see p. A-1) assigns a "3" or a "4" to combined contraceptive use in women with multiple risk factors for CAD. This means that the more risk factors a woman has, the more her risks may outweigh benefits from using estrogen.

MENOPAUSE: The permanent cessation of spontaneous menses, at an average age 51-52, creates an excellent opportunity to encourage healthy diets, exercise and health-promoting lifestyles (smoking cessation, calcium supplementation, etc.). Perhaps the single most important lifestyle message is that women who smoke as little as 1-4 cigarettes/day have a 2.5 fold increased risk of fatal coronary artery disease *[Speroff - 1999, p. 649]*

Common Physiologic Changes After Menopause

- Hot flashes/sleep disturbances, mood swings, decreased ability to concentrate and remember
- Thinning of genital urinary tissue (atrophic vaginitis, urinary incontinence)
- Osteopenia, osteoporosis, increased risk for fracture
- Increased risk for cardiovascular disease, unfavorable lipid profiles
- Increased risk of Alzheimer's disease, colon cancer, tooth loss, macular degenerative eye disease, decreased collagen and skin wrinkling, decreased short-term memory

HORMONE THERAPY (HRT, HT or ERT): A woman may choose to take hormones for short-term symptom relief and then reconsider that decision later. Each woman should be informed of potential benefits and risks of hormone replacement therapy.

HRT relieves vasomotor symptoms (hot flashes, night sweats) but is also used as preventive Rx to reduce some of the long term sequelae of estrogen deficiency: increased risk of vertebral, radial and femoral head fracture, and genital atrophy. 60% of females between the ages of 55-64 are sexually active. HRT (estrogen) helps alleviate decreased lubrication and genital atrophy.

The results of the widely publicized Women's Health Initiative study on combination HRT *[Writing Group WHI-2002]* has changed the landscape of prescribing HRT. The conclusion of the study states "Results from WHI indicate that the combined postmenopausal hormones CEE, 0.625 mg/d, plus MPA, 2.5 mg/d should not be initiated or continued for the primary prevention of CHD. In addition, the increased relative risks for CVD and breast CA (very small increased attributable risks) must be weighed against the benefit for reduction in fracture risk, reduction in colorectal cancer risk, relief of menopausal symptoms in selecting from the available agents." This randomized trial quantifies the increased relative risk women taking conjugated equine estrogen (CEE 0.625)/MPA 2.5 mg face: invasive breast CA 1.26, coronary heart disease 1.29, stroke 1.41 and pulmonary embolism. Other steroids and other routes of administration (transdermal and intrauterine) may alter the risk-benefit ratio

The focus today is to provide hormone therapy at the lowest possible dose for the shortest period of time only in symptomatic women

In March 2004, the estrogen-only arm of the WHI study was stopped because of an 8/10,000 increased risk for stroke

PRESCRIBING PRECAUTIONS FOR HRT
• Pregnancy; undiagnosed abnormal vaginal bleeding; active liver disease
• Recent or active thrombophlebitis or thromboembolic disorders (unless anticoagulated)
• Breast cancer or known or suspected estrogen-dependent neoplasm
• Recent myocardial infarction or severe cardiac artery disease

STARTING HORMONES FOR MENOPAUSAL WOMEN
• Patient counseling is key to success with HRT. Clearly describe onset of action of HRT for women with hot flashes as well as side effects (especially vaginal spotting and bleeding)
• Answer all questions about risks including a slightly increased risk for breast cancer, deep vein thrombosis, pulmonary embolism and cardiovascular disease *[WHI-2002]*
• Recent routine history and examination sufficient to identify any contraindications.
• Usual well-women care measures (e.g. mammogram, pap smear, lipid profile, thyroid function tests) should be provided but are not essential prior to starting HRT. Endometrial biopsy not needed except when evaluating abnormal vaginal bleeding
• Re-evaluate need for HRT/ERT/HT/HPT annually. The current products are:

Generic names - Estrogens	Brand names
Conjugated estrogen tablets, USP	Premarin®
Synthetic conjugated estrogens, A tablets	Cenestin®
Esterified estrogens tablets	Estratab®, Menest®
Estropipate tablets	Ogen®, Ortho-est®
Estradiol tablets	Estrace®
Matrix estradiol transdermal systems	Alora®, Climara®, FemPatch®, Vivelle™, Esclim, Menostar, Vivelle-dot
Reservoir estradiol transdermal systems	Estraderm®

Generic names - Progestins	Brand names
Medroxyprogesterone acetate (MPA) tablets	Amen®, Curretab®, Cycrin®, Provera®
Megestrol acetate tablets	Megace®
Norethindrone tablets	Micronor®, Nor-QD®, Norlutin®
Norethindrone acetate tablets	Aygestin®
Micronized progesterone capsules	Prometrium®
Progesterone vaginal gel	Crinone®
Levonorgestrel IUD	Mirena®

Generic names - Combined Products	Brand names
Estradiol and norgestimate tablets	Prefest®
Conjugated estrogens and MPA tablets	Premphase®, Prempro®
Esterified estrogens and methyl testosterone tablets	Estratest®, Estratest® H.S.
Ethinyl estradiol and norethindrone acetate tablets	Femhrt®
Estradiol and norethindrone tablets	Activella™
Matrix estradiol/ norethindrone acetate transdermal systems	CombiPatch™

FOLLOW-UP
• Be available to answer questions when there are media reports about HRT
• Patient should return in 1-3 months to answer further questions/manage side effects
• Have the woman keep a menstrual calendar of any breakthrough bleeding or spotting
• If hot flashes continue, consider thyroid dysfunction and other causes before increasing dose or using other therapeutic approaches to hotflash treatment

*Women in the reproductive years should be taking in 0.4 mg or 400 micrograms
of synthetic folic acid daily (whether pregnant or not).*
- *Every woman*
- *Every day*
- *400 micrograms of folic acid*

Assess:
- Reproductive, family and personal medical and surgical history with attention to pelvic surgeries
- Smoking, drug use, alcohol use: advise to stop and refer for help if needed
- Nutrition habits: identify excesses and inadequacies
- Medications: make adjustments in those that may affect fertility and/or pregnancy outcome. Advise patient not to make any changes without clinician's knowledge
- Risk for sexually transmitted infection/infertility in both partners
- Impacts of any medications (over-the-counter, prescription, herbal). For example, Accutane and tetracycline (which are teratogenic) for acne requires extremely effective contraception and strong consideration of the use of 2 contraceptives correctly. Advise ◄— that patient delay pregnancy for at least one year after last Accutane. See p. 38

Offer Screening for:
- Infections (TB, gonorrhea, chlamydia, HIV, syphilis, hepatitis B & C, HSV as per CDC guidelines). Vaginal wet mount if discharge present
- Neoplasms (breast, cervical dysplasia, warts, etc.)
- Immunity (rubella, tetanus, chicken pox, HBV)

Provide Genetic Counseling:
- For all women, but may need additional specialized counseling if going to be $\geq$ 35 y.o. when she delivers or has a significant personal or family history of genetic disorders, poor pregnancy outcome or multiple pregnancy ◄—
- Previous poor pregnancy outcomes
- Family history of mental retardation or genetic disorders such as sickle cell anemia, thalassemia, cystic fibrosis, Tay-Sachs, Canavan disease, neural tube defect
- High risk ethnic backgrounds - African Americans, Ashkenazi Jews, etc.
- Alcohol use, tobacco use, substance abuse
- Seizure disorders
- Diabetes, neural tube defects
- Other heritable medical problems

Assess Environmental Hazards:
- Chemical, radioactive and infectious exposures at workplace, home, hobbies
- Physical conditions, especially workplace

Assess Psychosocial Factors:
- Readiness of woman and partner for parenthood
- Mental health (depression, etc.) and domestic violence
- Financial issues and support systems

Recommend:

- ***Ideally, planning a pregnancy should involve both a woman and her partner***
- Balanced diet
- Do not eat shark, swordfish, mackerel, tilefish ←
- Eat up to 12 oz (2 coverage meals) of fish lower in mercury, which can include up to ← 6 oz of albacore tuna per week
- Vitamin with 0.4 mg folic acid for all women (use higher dose folic acid, 4 mg, in higher-risk women such as women with previous pregnancy with a neural tube defect, alcoholic, malabsorption or on anticonvulsants)
- Minimize STI exposure risk
- Weight loss, if obese (gradual loss until conception)
- Moderate exercise
- Avoiding exposure to cat feces (toxoplasmosis)
- Early in process of discussing pregnancy encourage breastfeeding as the best way to feed her baby

Avoid

- Raw meat (including fish) and unpasteurized dairy products
- Abdominal/pelvic X-rays, if possible
- Excesses in diet, vitamins, exercise
- Non-foods (pica), unusual herbs
- **Sex with multiple partners or sex with a partner who may be HIV-positive, have other STI or have other sex partner(s).** Use condom if any question. The possibility of a couple planning to become pregnant when one or both are having intercourse outside that relationship is an unfortunate reality. Condoms are not the answer to non-monogamy, but should be used in this case to protect the baby, the mother and the father. **Offer condoms to each pregnant woman** ←

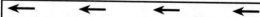

Here's a tip for people who have used this book in the past: in one or two hours you can find the major changes in the 2005-2007 edition. Simply thumb through the pages looking for the arrows! This would also be an excellent way to give a lecture on "what's new in family planning."

Early testing gives a woman a head start to pursue pregnancy options
- Prenatal care can be initiated promptly for the woman planning to keep the baby or give it up for adoption
- Ectopic pregnancies may be detected earlier
- Medical or surgical method of abortion, in part depending on gestational age

PREGNANCY TESTS

Urine tests:
- *Enzyme-linked immunosorbent assay (ELISA) test:*
  - Immunometric test uses antibody specific to placentally-produced HCG and another antibody to produce a color change. Commonly used in home pregnancy test and in offices and clinics. Performed in 1-3 minutes using urine samples
  - Most tests positive at levels of 25 mIU/ml. This level can be detectable 7-10 days after conception. May require 5-7 days after implantation to detect all pregnancies
  - Urine pregnancy tests are used in most clinical settings and are available for women to purchase over-the-counter; teach patients that no lab test is 100% accurate and that false negative tests (tests read as negative when a woman actually is pregnant) usually occur when done too early in the pregnancy and are far more common than false positive tests (tests read as positive when a woman actually is NOT pregnant)
  - 29 one-step urine tests sensitive to 10-25 mIU/ml beta hCG are outlined in table 26-2 on pages 636 and 637 of 18th edition of *Contraceptive Technology*. *"With a urine test kit with a sensitivity of 25 mIU/ml, results are positive for some women as early as 3-4 days after implantation (10 days after fertilization), test results are positive for 98% of women within 7 days after implantation." [Stewart in Contraceptive Technology, 2004]*

Serum tests (blood drawn):
- *Radioimmunoassay:*
  - Uses colorimetry, which detects HCG levels as low as 5 mIU/ml
  - Results available in 1-2 hours
  - Offers ability to quantify levels of HCG to monitor levels over time when clinically indicated

HCG QUICK FACTS
- β-HCG can be detected as early as 7-10 days after conception thereby, "ruling in" pregnancy, but pregnancy cannot be "ruled out" until 7 days after expected menses
- If needed for evaluation of early pregnancy, serial testing should be done every 2 days until levels reach discriminatory levels of 1800-2000 mIU/ml, when a gestational sac can be visualized reliably by vaginal ultrasound. In normal gestations the levels of HCG double about every 2 days *[Stenchever MA-2001]*
- Average time for HCG levels to become non-detectable after first trimester surgical abortion ranges from 31-38 days

MANAGEMENT TIPS
- Home tests can be misused or misinterpreted.
- Any test can have false-negative results at low levels. If in doubt, repeat urine test in 1-2 days or obtain serum tests with a qualitative HCG
- Folic acid, 0.4 mg/day: every woman, every day (pregnancy test positive or negative)

PREGNANCY TEST NEGATIVE: A TEACHABLE MOMENT

A negative pregnancy test for a woman not wanting to become pregnant clearly provides the counselor or clinician with a teachable moment and a time to offer a woman a better contraceptive and ECPs for future acts of intercourse that might be unprotected.

"Phew! The pregnancy test is negative." This must have been scary to worry that you might be pregnant.

1. If you haven't been using contraception, this is your "wake-up call." What contraceptive method would work best for you now? You may be able to start your contraceptive without a pelvic exam. ◄
2. Abstinence may be your chosen path now; if not, use contraception unless you want to become pregnant. Give her contraception now. Don't make her wait for another appointment. We can start most contraceptives without a pelvic exam.
3. Learn about emergency contraceptive pills and emergency IUD insertion.
4. Don't try to become pregnant in order to see if you can become pregnant.
5. Don't take a chance from this moment on: never, just never, have intercourse without knowing that you are protected against both infection and unintended or unwanted pregnancy.
6. Remember, your negative urine pregnancy test does not rule out conception from acts of intercourse in the past 2 weeks.
7. Provide emergency contraceptive pills (advance provision works).

PREGNANCY TEST POSITIVE: A TEACHABLE MOMENT

The pregnancy test is positive and she wants to continue the pregnancy. Whether or not this pregnancy was planned and prepared for,* your patient's mind is made up: she will continue this pregnancy, providing you, the counselor or clinician, with a teachable moment.

The pregnancy test is positive and she has definitely decided to continue her pregnancy to term

1. Start vitamins containing folic acid (0.4 mg) today. Buy vitamins on the way home. ALL WOMEN IN REPRODUCTIVE YEARS SHOULD BE ON FOLIC ACID
2. Stop drinking alcohol or using any illegal drugs today.
3. Stop smoking today.
4. Ask: "Are you on any medication?" ◄
5. Use condoms if at any risk for HIV or other STIs.
6. Eat healthy foods. Gain 25-30 pounds during your pregnancy (if your weight is now normal).
7. Review current medical problems.

* If she doesn't want to continue pregnancy, discuss pregnancy termination options or refer her to someone who feels comfortable doing this. Also discuss giving baby up for adoption

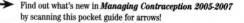

➤ Find out what's new in *Managing Contraception 2005-2007* by scanning this pocket guide for arrows!

Planning for postpartum (PP) contraception should begin during pregnancy and use should be initiated as early as possible postpartum. A newborn can place many demands on a woman's time, so her method should be as convenient for her to use as possible. In some women who are not consistently breastfeeding, ovulation may return within 3-6 weeks postpartum (before a woman realizes she is at risk which may well be before her first period). Involve partner as often as possible. Advance provision of EC is always appropriate ◄

AT DELIVERY
- Tubal sterilization may be performed (at C-section or after vaginal delivery)
- IUD may be inserted within 20 minutes of delivery of placenta (requires learning new technique) but rates of expulsion are higher than with insertion after uterine involution ◄

PRIOR TO LEAVING HOSPITAL
- Breastfeeding should be encouraged. Reinforce education about lactational amenorrhea if patient interested (see Chapter 15, p. 45-49)
- Pelvic rest (no douching, no sex, no tampons) is generally recommended for 4-6 weeks. Many women choose NOT to follow this advice in spite of increased risk for infection. Some clinicians encourage women to become sexually active when they feel comfortable and ready
- Women are strongly advised to abstain from intercourse until lochia has stopped
- At this time, sex may be the last thing the woman is thinking about. Nevertheless, encourage her to have a contraceptive plan for when she does intiate sexual activity. Options:
  - Tubal sterilization
  - Progestin-only methods: Depo-Provera (DMPA), progestin-only (mini) pills (POPs)
    NOTE: There are three approaches to starting these progestin-only methods: 1) When the patient leaves the hospital have her start oral iron if her hemoglobin is low and start POPs or DMPA; 2) Since progestin-only methods may prolong bleeding wait 2-3 weeks to start them (no data). Women with history of or high risk for postpartum depression may also benefit from a delay in starting progestin-only methods. In breastfeeding women, ◄ progestin-only methods have no effect on milk production or composition or long-term growth of the infant *(Cochrane Review presented at ARHP) (Truit-2003)*
  - Male or female condoms to reduce risk of sexually transmitted infections
  - Estrogen containing contraceptive may be prescribed for nonlactating women to start 3 weeks postpartum (risk of thrombosis associated with pregnancy reduced by that time). Recommend to start the Sunday after 21st day PP. Can give the woman a prescription when she leaves the hospital (to be started in 3 weeks)

AT POSTPARTUM VISIT (2-6 WEEKS)

- Ask if woman has resumed sexual intercourse
- Support continued breastfeeding
- Lactational amenorrhea follow-up. Provide condoms as transitional method prn return of menses, decrease in breastfeeding, etc
- Emergency contraception may be given if needed. PLAN B is most effective ECP
- Progestin-only methods may be provided (Depo-Provera, progestin-only pills, Mirena). Provide back-up method as needed if initiated when not on menses
- COCs, patch, ring or combined injectables may be started unless woman is exclusively breastfeeding. Provide backup method as needed
- IUD may be inserted if uterus well involuted (whether or not she is breast-feeding)
- Condoms (male or female) may be given as primary or backup contraceptive to provide STI risk reduction; withdrawal can be used at any time
- Tubal sterilization may be provided after uterine involution
- Diaphragm, cervical cap may be fitted after pelvis/cervix return to normal configuration
- NFP and FAM should await resumption of normal cycles

To order this book or *Contraceptive Technology*,
call (706) 265-7435 or go to www.managingcontraception.com
Excellent chapter on **Postpartum Contraception and Lactation**
by Kathy Irene Kennedy and James Trussell.

CHAPTER 12

Elective Abortion
www.prochoice.org/naf or www.earlyoptionpill.com

OVERVIEW

The availability of safe elective abortion procedures is important for fertility control; 48% of pregnancies in this country are unintended.

Surgical abortion techniques (especially uterine aspiration) have a proven safety profile, with serious morbidity in less than 1% of procedures and a death rate of 0.5/100,000 abortions (compared to maternal mortality with a continued pregnancy of approximately 7.3/100,000 deliveries). The introduction of several agents for early medical abortion have added new options.

Despite having one of the highest abortion rates among developed countries, in 2000, over 78% of US counties had no abortion providers or facilities. It is now up to 87%. Many state laws impose mandatory restrictions, waiting periods, and consent requirements. For current information on your state's abortion laws, contact Pro Choice America 202-973-3000 or www.naral.org/). Approximately 1.3 million abortions are performed in the U.S. each year; 88% are first trimester and 97% are surgical. By 2000, approximately 80,000 medical abortions were provided in the U.S. [Hausknect-2003]

The pattern of induced abortions in the United States has changed from 1994 to 2000:
• The likelihood of a reproductive age woman having an abortion fell 11%
• Abortions among 15-17 year old women fell 39%
• Abortions among 18-19 year olds fell 18%
• Abortions for women at less than 100% above poverty increased 25%
• Abortions for women at 100-199% above poverty level increased 23%
• **In 2000, 25% of all pregnancies ended in an induced abortion.** [Jones-2002]

Features of Medical Compared to Surgical Abortion

Medical	Surgical
Generally avoids invasive procedure	Involves invasive procedure
Requires multiple visits	Usually requires one visit
Days to weeks until complete	Usually complete in a few minutes
Available during very early pregnancy	Available during early and later pregnancy
High success rate (94% - 97%)	Higher success rate (99%)
Requires follow-up to ensure completion of abortion	Does not require follow-up in most cases
May be more private in some circumstances; will vary for each individual patient	May be more private in some circumstances; will vary for each individual patient
Patient participation in multi-step process	Less patient participation in a single-step process
	Allows use of sedation or anesthesia if desired
Does not require surgical training	Requires surgical training and sometimes licensed facility

31

ELECTIVE SURGICAL ABORTION

DESCRIPTION
Voluntary termination of pregnancy using uterine aspiration in early intrauterine gestations. In later gestations (after 14 weeks) use instruments for tissue removal (dilation and extraction, D & E).

EFFECTIVENESS
- 98-99% effective; failures are mostly incomplete abortions with small amounts of retained tissue; rarely does the pregnancy continue

PROCEDURE
- After informed consent obtained according to local law, type of procedure is determined by gestational age and patient preference
- In second trimester, dilate the cervix with an osmotic dilator such as laminaria OR with a prostaglandin analogue such as misoprostol with or without laminaria ◄
- Antibiotic prophylaxis reduces risk of post-procedure infection.
  Doxycycline 200 mg 30-60 minutes prior to and immediately after procedure or metronidazole 1 g preoperatively and 500 mg orally every 6 hours for 3 doses.
  If chlamydia infection likely, a 7-day course of doxycycline, or a single dose of ◄ azithromycin 1 g may be given. If BV is present, treat systemically with p.o. antibiotics
- Cleanse ectocervix and endocervix
- Administer cervical anesthesia; if desired, adjunctive sedation can also be used. NSAIDS are administered by some clinicians
- Place tenaculum and mechanically dilate cervix if not previously dilated adequately
- Using sterile technique, insert a plastic cannule and apply suction to aspirate products of conception either with a machine, or manually with a syringe (in MVA-manual uterine aspiration)
- May confirm adequacy of procedure by checking uterine cavity with a sharp curette (optional)
- Evaluate tissue to confirm presence of placental villi/gestational sac if early pregnancy. If more than 9 weeks should be able to visualize fetal tissue
- Administer Rh immune globulin if woman is Rh negative

ADVANTAGES
- Provides woman complete control over her fertility
- Ability to prevent an unwanted or defective birth or halt a pregnancy that poses risk to maternal health or other aspects of her life that she deems important
- Safe and rapid; preoperative evaluation and procedure can usually be done in a single visit from a medical perspective (local legal restrictions may affect this)
- No increase in risk of breast cancer, infertility, cervical incompetence, preterm labor, or congenital anomalies in subsequent pregnancy after uncomplicated first-trimester abortion
- Safer for maternal health than continuing pregnancy
- Can be provided as early as intrauterine pregnancy is diagnosed

DISADVANTAGES
- Most women experience cramping and pain with procedure; the noise of the vacuum machine (if electrical vacuum used) may cause anxiety. (Manual vacuum aspiration or MVA may be more tolerable for this reason)
- Possibility of later regret (regret is equally possible for undesired pregnancy that is continued)

COMPLICATIONS

• Infection <1%, with an uncommon complication of infertility
• Incomplete abortion 0.5%-1.0%; Failed abortion 0.1%-0.5%
• Missed ectopic pregnancy is possible. Check evacuated tissue for presence of chorionic villi ◄
• Hemorrhage 0.03%-1.0%
• Post-abortal syndrome (hematometra) <1%
• Asherman's syndrome rare (more likely with septic abortion), with an uncommon complication of infertility
• Mortality: Elective abortion deaths <1 per 100,000 (compared to pregnancy deaths/childbirth 7.3/100,000) (Safer than pregnancy or tonsilectomy)

CANDIDATES FOR USE

• Any woman requesting abortion. State laws often limit gestational age (typically available through 24 weeks). State laws may also affect access and consent procedures
Adolescents: State laws vary regarding requirements and consent requirements (See p. 19)

INITIATING METHOD

• Carefully discuss all pregnancy options, including prenatal care for parenting or for adoption and programs available for assistance with each option
• If patient chooses abortion, discuss available techniques when applicable (surgical versus medical)
• Obtain informed consent after answering all questions
• Offer emotional support, education, pre- and post-procedural instructions, and contraception
• Usually perform procedure in outpatient setting unless woman has severe medical problems requiring more intense monitoring or deeper anesthesia
• Initiate contraception immediately after procedure

INSTRUCTIONS

• Keep telephone number(s) nearby for any emergencies
• May resume usual activities same day if procedure done under local anesthesia
• One week pelvic rest (no tampons, douching or sexual intercourse)
• Use NSAIDs or acetaminophen for cramping, NSAIDs or ergotamine (methergine) for bleeding
• Showers are permitted immediately ◄
• Seek medical care urgently if heavy bleeding, excessive cramping, pain, fevers, chills, or malodorous discharge
• After 1 week of abstinence, use contraception with every single act of intercourse and keep EC available for future use

FOLLOW-UP

• Have you had a temperature >100.4°F?
• What has your bleeding been like since the procedure?
• Have you had any new abdominal or pelvic pain?
• Do you plan to have children? OR When do you plan to have more children?
• Are you using a contraceptive?

PROBLEM MANAGEMENT

Infection

- Always evaluate possibility of retained products and need for reaspiration
- Patients who develop endometritis can generally be treated using outpatient PID therapies described in the CDC Guidelines (see Chapter 31 p. 165)
- Cases that are more complicated may require hospitalization and IV antibiotics (rare)

Persistent or excessive bleeding

- *Possible causes* : uterine atony, retained products, uterine perforation, cervical laceration
- *Treat likely cause(s)*: Use uterine-contracting agents for atony (methergine, hemabate, misoprostol). Reaspirate if retained products. If uterine perforation, give antibiotics, and evaluate surgically if there is concern for bowel or vascular injury. Suture external cervical lacerations; tamponade endocervical lacerations
- *For significant hemorrhage (rare)*: transfuse if large blood loss. Provide blood factors to patients with coagulopathies. In extremely rare cases, uterine atery embolization, ⬅ further surgery or hysterectomy may be necessary

ELECTIVE MEDICAL ABORTION

DESCRIPTION

- The first medication (mifepristone or methotrexate) is given to interrupt the further development of the pregnancy
- Misoprostol is then given to induce expulsion of the products of conception
- Misoprostol is a prostaglandin analogue which causes the cervix to soften and the uterus to contract. May be taken orally or vaginally, either at home or in the office. (Not as effective when given alone as when given with either mifepristone or methotrexate) *[Goldberg, Greenberg, and Darney-NEJM 2001]*

INITIATING METHOD

- Discuss all pregnancy options, including prenatal care for parenting or for adoption and highlight programs available for assistance with each option
- If patient chooses elective abortion, discuss available techniques (surgical vs. medical)
- Review protocol, risks, benefits, and visit schedule
- Assess patient's access to provider if D&C is needed. Explain need for D&C if incomplete or if continuing pregnancy (some women think they can avoid surgery altogether) ⬅
- Obtain informed consent after all questions are answered
- Vaginal ultrasound to confirm dates if available

MEDICAL ABORTION WITH MIFEPRISTONE (RU-486) AND MISOPROSTOL (MIS)

Most medical abortions in the U.S. and abroad now use mifepristone rather than methotrexate. RU-486 used as an abortifacient in France since 1988 and in other European countries and China.

Mechanism - Mifepristone acts as an antiprogesterone to block continued support of the pregnancy. It blocks progesterone receptors. This causes decidual necrosis and detachment of products of conception. Mifepristone also causes cervical softening

Dose - 600 mg is FDA approved dose - but 200 mg is just as effective in clinical trials

Effectiveness - 94-97% effective depending on gestational age and MIS doses used: for gestational age up to 49 days if using oral MIS, up to 63 days if vaginal MIS. Process is generally more rapid than if using methotrexate and MIS

Contraindications - Not effective for ectopics. Use MTX if suspicious for ectopic. Not for use by chronic corticosteroid users, chronic adrenal failures, porphyrias, or with history of allergy to RU-486 or prostaglandins

Protocol - (adapted from National Abortion Federation Guidelines)

- **Day 1:** Baseline labs including blood type with Rh, hemoglobin. Rh immunoglobin if Rh negative. Give mifepristone 200 mg orally
- **Day 2 or 3:** MIS 800 ug into posterior fornix of vagina (usually 4 x 200 ug tabs - some clinicians have found they are more efffective when moistened with saline or water)
- **Day 15:** Assess expulsion; pelvic exam, ultrasound (if needed). For heavy bleeding, signs of infection or failed abortion, perform D&C, offer observation or repeat MIS if only tissue present (not fetus) and return appointment in 2-4 weeks

MEDICAL ABORTION WITH METHOTREXATE (MTX) AND MISOPROSTOL (MIS)

Mechanism - Methotrexate is administered to prevent continued implantation of the pregnancy. It prevents reduction of folic acid to tetrahydrofolate by binding to dihydrofolate reductase. This prevents proliferation of placental villi by interfering with DNA synthesis

Dose - 50 mg/m^2 IM or 50 mg PO

Effectiveness - 94-96% effective up to 49 days gestational age (rates drop to 84% if 50-56 days). 15-20% of women have 20-30 day delay in abortion and bleeding. Therapeutic for ectopic pregnancies in 90-95% of cases

Contraindications - not for women with kidney or liver dysfunction. <1% of women will develop neutropenia, stomatitis, or oral ulcers from the MTX

Protocol - (adapted from National Abortion Federation Guidelines)

- **Day 1:** Baseline labs including blood type with Rh, hemoglobin (liver function tests and creatinine, if clinically indicated). MTX 50 mg/m^2 body surface area IM or 50 mg orally. Rh immunoglobin if Rh negative
- **Day 6 or 7:** MIS 800 ug into posterior fornix of vagina (usually 4 x 200 ug tabs - some clinicians have found they are more efffective when moistened with saline or water)
- **Day 15:** Assess expulsion; pelvic exam, ultrasound (if needed). For heavy bleeding, signs of infection, or failed abortion, perform D&C. Offer observation or repeat MIS if only tissue present (not fetus) and return appointment in 2-4 weeks

ADVANTAGES

- Provides a women with more reproductive choices
- Very early abortions can be performed
- Potentially private
- Less risk of operative complications (risk only if aspiration required)
- Some women feel more in control of the precess, feel it is more "natural"
- Provides option to women who may not have access to surgical options as readily (although need to have provider available to perform D&C if needed)

DISADVANTAGES

- Abdominal cramping, nausea (3-61%), vomiting (2-26%), diarrhea (3-20%), fever and chills (7-60%)
- Heavy vaginal bleeding after the misoprostol is taken. May need to provide prolonged access to bathroom facilties if patients observed in office or clinic after misoprostol is given
- Vaginal bleeding averages 10-17 days
- Methotrexate and misoprostol are teratogenic drugs; follow-up is essential to assure that the abortion is complete

COMPLICATIONS

- Ongoing pregnancy (with exposure to potential teratogen) (<1%)
- Incomplete abortion requiring surgical curettage (most failures are for incomplete abortions)
- Hemorrhage requiring emergent curettage
- Approximately 5% will require surgical D&C for one of the preceeding three reasons
- Infection (<1%)
- Blood transfusion if significant hemorrhage (<2/100,000) *[Hausknecht-2003]*

CANDIDATES FOR USE

- Pregnant women, well dated by LMP and/or ultrasound, desiring medical termination of pregnancy
- Women willing to comply with instructions and visit schedule until procedure complete
- Women who are not anemic, have coagulation disorders, or are on anticoagulants

INSTRUCTIONS FOR PATIENT

- Expect moderate (occasionally severe) cramping, bleeding, and nausea
- Call or seek help if heavy bleeding (soaking 4 sanitary pads within 2 hours)
- Abstain from sexual intercourse, alcohol, vitamins, or folate supplements during treatment
- Either return for misoprostol or take it at home as directed
- Use acetaminophen or NSAID's for analgesia; use codeine if inadequate relief
- Have a support person/emergency plan available after misoprostol given

PROBLEM MANAGEMENT

Pain - oral analgesics, including NSAIDs, 1/300 women need IV analgesia *[Creinin-1997]*
Bleeding - D&C done for hemorrhage or anemia requiring transfusion (occurs 1/1000)
Nausea/vomiting/diarrhea/fever - use over-the-counter antiemetics, Lomotil, acetaminophen; drink fluids

FERTILITY AFTER USE

- Immediate return to baseline fertility. Contraceptive should be supplied immediately
- No evidence of harm in future pregnancies due to these medications

EARLY MEDICAL ABORTION WITH MISOPROSTOL ALONE

Misoprostol is a prostaglandin analogue which causes very strong uterine contractions and can terminate pregnancy after 2-3 doses of 400-800 micrograms each

- Studies with misoprostol alone show efficacy of 68-94% up to 49 days, only 47-88% up to 56 days
- Given the inconsistency of complete abortion rates when vaginal misoprostol is used alone, as well as the existence of safe alternative regimens, it generally is not recommended for medical abortions in the first trimester *[Goldberg, Greenberg and Darney - NEJM Jan 2001]*

CHAPTER 13

Choosing Among Available Methods
www.managingcontraception.com/choices
www.plannedparenthood.org/library

THE BEST METHOD IS THE ONE THAT IS MEDICALLY APPROPRIATE AND IS USED EVERY TIME BY SOMEONE HAPPY WITH THE METHOD

- Be aware of your own biases
- Each contraceptive method has both advantages and disadvantages
- Effectiveness and safety are important (see Tables 13.2, p. 39 and 13.3, p. 40)
- Convenience and ability to use method correctly influences effectiveness
- Protection against STIs/HIV needs to be considered for women and men at risk
- Effects of method on menses may be very important to a woman
- Ability to negotiate with partner may help determine method selected
- Religion, privacy, friend's advice and frequency of sex may influence decision
- Discuss all methods with patient, even those you may not use in your own practice
- Is partner supportive of contraception/condoms and will he help pay for them?
- Consider discussing with couple, particularly if there appears to be conflict

EFFECTIVENESS: measured by failure rates in 2 ways (see Table 13.2, p. 39)
Correct and consistent use first year failure rate: The percentage of women who become pregnant during their first year of use when they use the method perfectly. ←
Typical use first year failure rates: The percentage of women who become pregnant during their first year of use. This number reflects pregnancies in couples who use the method correctly and consistently and of those who do not. **This typical use failure rate is the relevant number to use when counseling new start users.**

- In spite of many very effective options, the U.S. has a high rate of unintended pregnancy. Just under 50% of all pregnancies in the U.S. are not planned. Our challenge is to help women and couples use more effectively already available methods

KEY QUESTIONS

- *What contraceptive did you come to this office today wanting to use?* Data show that giving the method they ask for is more likely to result in continuation. *[Pariani S. et al. Stud Fam Plann, 1991]* ←
- *Do you plan to have children? OR Do you plan to have more children?*
  If she says she definitely wants no further pregnancies, be sure to discuss sterilization in addition to the highly effective reversible methods.
- *When (if ever) do you want to have your next child?*
  Helps teach need for preconceptional care and guides in selection of method
- *Does your partner want to have children in the future? When?*
- *What would you do if you had an accidental pregnancy? Is abortion an option or not?* Provide ECPs and discuss use of 2 methods ←
- *What method(s) did you use in the past? What problems did you have with it/them?* ←
- *What are you doing to protect yourself from STIs/AIDS?*
  Inclusion of counseling about safer sex practices and condoms may be critical

- *Would you like to learn about emergency contraception?*

  Would she like a package of ECPs or a prescription for ECPs?

- *Do you have any serious medical problems?*

TABLE 13.1 Comparative risk of unprotected intercourse on unintended pregnancies and STI infections*

Unintended pregnancy/coital act	PID per woman infected with cervical gonorrhea
17%-30% midcycle	40% if not treated
<1% during menses	0% if promptly and adequately treated
Gonococcal transmission/coital act	**Tubal infertility per PID episode**
50% infected male, uninfected female	8% after first episode
25% infected female, uninfected male	20% after second episode
	40% after three or more episodes

*Cates W Jr. Reproductive tract infections. In: Hatcher RA, et al. Contraceptive Technology. 17th ed. New York: Ardent Media, 1998:181.

Should Accutane (isotretinoin) be withheld from young reproductive-age women? No, but it should certainly be used very cautiously

Accutane (isotretinoin) is a vitamin A isomer used in the treatment of extremely severe acne. Try to avoid its use. Use only if acne is severe. If taken by a woman who is pregnant, it may cause a wide range of teratogenic effects from:

CNS: hydrocephalus, facial nerve palsy, cortical blindness and retinal defects AND

Craniofacial: low-set ears, microcephaly, triangular skull and cleft palate to

Cardiovascular: transposition of the great vessels, atrial and ventricular septal defects

Important contraceptive messages for women considering Accutane use, in view of the fact that no method of birth control is 100% effective:

- **Use Two Methods:** In addition to compulsively careful and consistent use of a very effective hormonal contraceptive or intrauterine device, also use condoms consistently and correctly. Use of any combined pill is likely to have a beneficial effect on acne.

- **Repeated Pregnancy Tests:** Pregnancy tests are essential prior to initiating and on a monthly basis thereafter. This is particularly important since the critical time of exposure to Accutane is believed to be 2-5 weeks after conception [Briggs-2002]

- **Consider Abortion if Contraceptive Failure:** Should pregnancy occur, strongly consider having an abortion performed. It is clear that this is happening. In the 22 months following its introduction, the manufacturer, FDA and CDC received reports on 154 Accutane-exposed pregnancies, of which 95 (61.7%) were electively aborted. Another 12 (7.8%) aborted spontaneously. 26 were born without major defects and 21 had major malformations [Briggs-2002] Many clinicians will not provide this drug unless the woman using it agrees to have an abortion should a pregnancy exposed to Accutane occur

- **Use Accutane Sparingly:** This drug is so dangerous to a developing fetus that it should not be used unless other approaches to managing acne have been used first AND unless the reproductive-age woman using it agrees to use two contraceptives consistently and correctly.

Table 13.2 Percentage of women experiencing an unintended pregnancy within the first year of typical use and the first year of perfect use and the percentage continuing use at the end of the first year: United States[*]

Method	% of Women Experiencing an Unintended Pregnancy within the First Year of Use		% of Women Continuing Use at One Year[1]
	Typical Use[2]	Perfect Use[3]	
No Method[4]	85	85	
Spermicides[5]	29	18	42
Withdrawal	27	4	43
Periodic Abstinence			51
Calendar	25	9	
Ovulation Method	25	3	
Symptothermal[6]	25	2	
Post-ovulation	25	1	
Cervical Cap with spermicide			
Parous Women	32	26	46
Nulliparous Women	16	9	57
Diaphragm with spermicide[7]	16	6	57
Condom[8]			
Reality Female Polyurethane condom	21	5	49
Male (Latex or polyurethane)	15	2	53
Pill (COCs and POPs)	8	0.3	68
Ortho Evra patch	8	0.3	68
NuvaRing	8	0.3	68
Depo-Provera injections - q.3 months	3	0.3	56
Lunelle monthly injection	3	0.05	56
IUD			
Copper T (Paragard)	0.8	0.6	78
Levonorgestrel-releasing (Mirena)	0.1	0.1	81
Female Sterilization	0.5	0.5	100
Male Sterilization	0.15	0.10	100

Emergency Contraceptive Pills: Treatment with COCs initiated within 120 hours after unprotected intercourse reduces the risk of pregnancy by at least 60-75%.[9] Pregnancy rates lower if initiated in first 12 hours. Progestin-only EC reduces pregnancy risk by 89%.
Lactational Amenorrhea Method: LAM is a highly effective, temporary method of contraception.[10]

[1] Among couples attempting to avoid pregnancy, the percentage who continue to use a method for 1 year
[2] Among typical couples who initiate use of a method (not necessarily for the first time), the percentage who experience an accidental pregnancy during the first year if they do not stop use for any other reason
[3] Among couples who initiate use of a method (not necessarily for the first time) and who use it perfectly (both consistently and correctly), the percentage who experience an accidental pregnancy during the first year if they do not stop use for any other reason
[4] The percentages becoming pregnant in columns 2 and 3 are based on data from populations where contraception is not used and from women who cease using contraception in order to become pregnant. Among such populations, about 89% become pregnant within 1 year. This estimate was lowered slightly (to 85) to represent the percentages who would become pregnant within 1 year among women now relying on reversible methods of contraception if they abandoned contraception altogether
[5] Foams, creams, gels, vaginal suppositories, and vaginal film
[6] Cervical mucus (ovulation) method supplemented by calendar in the pre-ovulatory and basal body temperature in the post-ovulatory phases
[7] With spermicidal cream or jelly
[8] With or without spermicides (No difference in efficacy)
[9] The treatment schedule is one dose within 72 hours after unprotected intercourse, and a second dose 12 hours after the first dose. See page 70 for pills that may be used
[10] However, to maintain effective protection against pregnancy, another method of contraception must be used as soon as menstruation resumes, the frequency or duration of breast-feedings is reduced, bottle feeds are introduced, or the baby reaches 6 months of age

[*] Adapted from Trussell J, Kowal D. The essentials of contraception. In: Hatcher RA, et al. *Contraceptive Technology*, 18th ed. New York: Ardent Media, 2004.

Implanon has not yet been added by Trussell. Darney's recommendation: Perfect use 0.0 and Typical use 0.1% ◄

Table 13.3 Major methods of contraception and some related safety concerns, side effects, and noncontraceptive benefits
*Trussell J, Kowal D. The essentials of contraception. IN: Hatcher RA, et al. *Contraceptive Technology*. 17th ed. New York: Ardent Media, 1998:235. Slight adaptations from CT table.

METHOD	NONCONTRACEPTIVE BENEFITS*	SIDE EFFECTS	COMPLICATIONS
Combined pills, injections, patch and ring	Decreased dysmenorrhea, PMS, and blood loss; protects against symptomatic PID requiring hospitalization, ovarian and endometrial carcinomas, some benign tumors (leiomyomata, benign breast masses), ectopic pregnancies and ovarian cysts; reduces acne	Nausea, vomiting, headaches, dizziness, mastalgia, chloasma, spotting and bleeding, mood changes including, depression (rare)	Cardiovascular complications (DVT, PE, MI, hypertension), severe depression, hepatic adenoma, slight increase in adenocarcinoma of cervix
Progestin-only pills	Lactation not disturbed. Decreased menstrual blood loss	Spotting, breakthrough bleeding, amenorrhea, mood changes, headaches, hot flashes	None
Progestin-only implants	Lactation not disturbed. Less blood loss per cycle. Reduced risk of ectopic pregnancy	Menstrual changes, mood changes, weight gain or loss, headaches, hair loss	Infection at implant site, reaction to anesthesia, complicated removal, depression
Progestin-only injections	Lactation not disturbed. Reduces risk of sickle cell crises, endometrial cancer, ovarian cysts, mittelschmerz. May reduce risk of PID, seizures, ovarian cancer. Can be used with anti-convulsants	Menstrual changes, weight gain, headaches, hair loss, adverse impact on lipids, mood changes including, severe depression (rare)	Allergic reaction, excessive weight gain, glucose intolerance, depression
IUD	Lactation not disturbed. Copper T & levonorgestrel IUDs reduce risk for ectopic preg. LNG IUD reduces cramping & pain & treats bleeding from DUB, menorrhagia, & fibroids	Copper-IUD increases menstrual flow, blood loss and cramping. LNG IUD may cause irregular bleeding/amenorrhea	PID following insertion, uterine perforation, bleeding with expulsion
Sterilization	Women: reduced risk of ovarian cancer, endometrial cancer, ectopic pregnancy, PID Men: none known	Pain at surgical site, adhesion formation, subsequent regret	Surgical complications: hemorrhage, infection, organ damage, anesthetic complications, pain, ectopic pregnancy
Abstinence	Prevents most STIs, cervical dysplasia; enhanced self-image possible	None except possible peer pressure; Partner may seek sex elsewhere	None known
Male latex condom	Reduces risk of STIs and cervical dysplasia	Decrease in spontaneity or sensation; allergic reaction to latex, skin irritation	Rare anaphylactic reactions to latex (use polyurethane condoms)
Female condom	May reduce STI and cervical dysplasia risk	Difficult to use, vaginal and bladder infection	Toxic shock syndrome (although no cases reported)
Diaphragm Cervical cap	Reduces risk of cervical STIs, PID and possibly cervical dysplasia	Vaginal and bladder infection, vaginal erosions from poorly fit device, allergy to spermicide/latex	Toxic shock syndrome, anaphylactic reaction to latex

TIMING:

Couples considering contraceptives and their health care providers face myriad questions about the timing of contraceptive use. Sometimes our clients come to us with mistaken ideas. Sometimes we providers are actually the source of arbitrary misinformation about timing. In either case, timing errors, misconceptions, rigidity and oversimplifications can cause trouble; and trouble in family planning often can be spelled unintended pregnancy. In most instances, more important than advice about the timing of contraceptives is rapid initiation and then correct, ***consistent*** use of contraceptives. Below are several suggestions to consider in helping patients with timing questions:

1. For many women, a practical way to start pills, the patch or the ring is on the first day of the next period. Even easier, sometimes, is the Quick Start method which is to start pills on the day you first see a patient if you can be reasonably certain that she is not pregnant *[Westhoff 2002]*. Recommend backup method for 7 days unless pills started during the five days after the start of menses or within 5 days of miscarriage. Women with unprotected intercourse in preceeding 5 days should also receive EC

2. Switching from one hormonal method to another can be done immediately as long as the first method is used consistently and correctly, or if it is reasonably certain that she is not pregnant

3. Healthy women who tolerate pills well and do not smoke can continue pills indefinitely or until menopause unless a woman develops a complication or a contraindication to pill use. Periodic "breaks" from taking pills, still recommended by some clinicians, is an unwise practice that can lead to unintended pregnancies

4. Extended use of combined pills with no pill free interval is an acceptable way for some women to take pills, with no increased risk of endometrial hyperplasia *[Anderson-2003]*

5. The first Depo-Provera injection may be given at any time in the cycle if a woman is not pregnant. If the day of the first shot is NOT within 5 days of the start of a period, recommend that patient use a back-up contraceptive for 7 days; give EC and repeat pregnancy test in 2-3 weeks if recent unprotected intercourse

6. Avoid overly dogmatic advice regarding when postpartum women should start progestin-only pills and the progestin-only injection, Depo-Provera. There are clinicians and entire programs starting these two methods in each of the following 3 ways:
   - At discharge from hospital
   - 3 weeks postpartum
   - 6 weeks postpartum

7. Recommend that condoms be placed onto the erect penis OR onto the penis before it becomes erect. There are clear advantages and disadvantages to both approaches.

8. Offer Plan B (emergency contraceptive pills) to women in advance. Advance prescription of Plan B is one approach. Better yet, hand her the actual pills and instructions

9. Intrauterine contraceptives may be inserted at any time in a woman's menstrual cycle if she is not pregnant. Backup recommended for 7 days if not inserted in first 7 days of cycle

10. If in doubt about any timing question, use condoms until your timing questions have been resolved

DESCRIPTION

Surveys reveal a wide variety of opinions about what constitutes sexual activity. However, from a family planning perspective, the definition of abstinence is clear: it is delaying genital contact that could result in a pregnancy (i.e. penile penetration into the vagina). Some authors argue that abstinence is not a form of contraception, but is a lifestyle choice because person delaying intercourse needs no contraception. Regardless, abstinence is an important means of reducing unintended pregnancies and sexually transmitted infections. ←
A woman or a man may return to abstinence at any time. Abstinence-only-until-marriage education programs receive more than $100 million annually in U.S. government funding, most of it stemming from the Personal Responsibility and Work Opportunity Reconciliation Act of 1996. There is currently little to no evidence that any of these programs, which promote sexual abstinence and restrict information about contraception, actually achieve their intended purposes. Recent data from the state of MN has shown an increase in teen sexual activity and pregnancy during the first four years of such a program

EFFECTIVENESS
Perfect use failure rate in first year: 0%
Typical use failure rates in first year: Unknown

MECHANISM
Sperm excluded from female reproductive tract, preventing fertilization

COST: None, except expense of pregnancy or pregnancy termination if plans change

ADVANTAGES: Can be restarted at any time!
Menstrual: none
Sexual/psychological:
  • Can increase self esteem and positive self image if consistent with personal values
  • Can increase communication, negotiation skills and confidence
Cancers, tumors, and masses:
  • Risk of cervical cancer far less if no vaginal intercourse has ever occurred
Other:
  • Reduces risk of STIs (varies by what other sexual practices involved)
  • Many religions and cultures endorse (at various stages in an individual's life)

DISADVANTAGES
Menstrual: None
Sexual/psychological: Frustration or sense of rejection if abstinence not self-selected
Cancers, tumors, and masses: None except indirectly. Virgins obviously remain nulliparous and, because of their nulliparity until an older age, have an increased risk for breast and ovarian cancer
Other:
  • Requires commitment and self control; nonunderstanding partner may seek other partner(s)
  • Patient and her partner may not be prepared to contracept if they stop abstaining

COMPLICATIONS
• No medical complications

- Person may be in situation where she/he wants to abstain, but partner does not agree. Women have been raped/beaten for refusing to have intercourse. Clearly, this is wrong. Occasionally there are dire consequences from the decision not to have intercourse.

CANDIDATES FOR USE
- Individuals or couples who feel they have ability to refrain from sexual intercourse

Adolescents:
  - Very appropriate method but need to learn negotiating skills to effectively use abstinence and obtain information about contraceptive methods for future
  - Counseling may include discussions on masturbation (solo or mutual) and also "outercourse" alternative ways of expressing affection/attraction/sexuality with partner

INITIATING METHOD USUALLY REQUIRES OPEN COMMUNICATION
- Provide negotiating skills, how to say no or "not now", and how to resist peer (societal) pressures
- Recommend that patient ensure that partner explicitly agrees to abstain
- Stress that abstinence may just be a decision to delay intercourse. It may mean "not now", instead of "never". Remind her that she may use or return to abstinence at any time in life

INSTRUCTIONS FOR PATIENT
- Establish ground rules for herself and partner
- Prepare for time when (or if) decision to stop abstaining arises, initiate contraceptive counseling now
- Encourage her to consider having condoms and emergency contraception on hand in case of need

PROBLEM MANAGEMENT
Partner does not want to abstain:
- Consider counseling in negotiating skills, role playing exercises and couple's counseling
- Provide counseling in other forms of sexual pleasuring if patient interested (masturbation or outercourse)
- Seriously consider another birth control method or another partner!

FERTILITY AFTER DISCONTINUATION OF METHOD
- Protects against upper reproductive tract infection preserving a woman's fertility

---

Are Abstinence-Only Education Programs Effective?

According to a recent literature review conducted by Kirby (2001) for the National Campaign to Prevent Teen Pregnancy, only three evaluation studies of abstinence-only programs met the criteria established for inclusion in the review (e.g. random assignment, large sample size, long-term follow-up, measurement of behavior). All three studies measured program impact on the initiation of sex or frequency of sex. **None of the studies demonstrated a significant programmatic effect on the initiation of sex, frequency of sexual activity, or the number of sexual partners.** Although the results are not encouraging based on these three studies, Kirby concludes that there is insufficient evidence that abstinence-only programs do or do not delay sexual behavior. Large-scale evaluation data of the federally funded abstinence-only programs that resulted from the 1996 welfare reform act are expected soon. ←

Source: Kirby, D. (2001). Emerging Answers: Research Findings on Programs to Reduce Teen Pregnancy. Washington, DC: The National Campaign to Prevent Teen Pregnancy.

WAYS TO ENCOURAGE ABSTINENCE ◄

Ways to Think About Abstinence

1. *Primary Abstinence* for a very long period of time - eg until marriage or until engaged.

2. *Return to Abstinence* for a very long time. Some call this **"secondary virginity"**

3. *Abstinence "for a while" - for example, until*
   a) effective contraception has been achieved or until
   b) STD tests are negative and effective approach to prevention of STDs carefully discussed
      and agreed upon by both partners or until
   c) 2, 4, or 6 week postpartum visit

4. *Abstinence right now - tonight or today.* We don't have a condom. We have any question
at all about contraception. Each night there are some 10 million acts of intercourse in couples
NOT wanting to become pregnant and 700,000 of those acts of intercourse are completely
unprotected acts of sexual intercourse. Tonight 700,000 couples could decide NOT to have
intercourse tonight.

Each of those 4 time frames for abstinence (avoiding penis-in-vagina intercourse) may or may
not be complimented by any of a variety of sexual interactions sometimes called **outercourse**
(holding hands, hugging, kissing, deep kissing, petting, mutual masturbation, oral-genital
contact).

CHAPTER 15

Breastfeeding: Lactational Amenorrhea Method (LAM)

www.lalecheleague.org or www.breastfeeding.com or www.ilca.org

DESCRIPTION: The lactational amenorrhea method (LAM) is
contingent upon nearly exclusive or exclusive, frequent breastfeeding.
LAM is an effective method only under specific conditions:

- Woman breast-feeding exclusively; both day and night feedings
  (at least 90% of baby's nutrition derived from breast-feeding)
- The woman is amenorrheic (spotting which occurs in the first 56 days
  postpartum is not regarded as menses)
- The infant is less than 6 months old

If you don't understand the numbers, you don't understand the enterprise: In the U.S.,
the median duration of breast-feeding is about 3 months. It is important to provide a woman
with another method to use when she no longer fulfills all the conditions. **The probability
that ovulation will precede the first menstrual period in a lactating woman increases from
33-45% during the first 3 months to 64-71% during months 4 to 12 and 87% after
12 months.** *[Kennedy K.I. IN Hatcher RA Contraceptive Technology 18th Edition]*. Among
lactating women, 66% are sexually active in the first month postpartum and 88% are
sexually active in the second month postpartum *[Ford - 1998]*

EFFECTIVENESS *[Kennedy - 1998]*
Perfect use failure rate in first 6 months: 0.5%
Typical use failure rate in first 6 months: 2%
At any time a woman is concerned, emergency contraception may be used by a nursing
mother (preferably with levonorgestrel-only pills - Plan B)

MECHANISM: Suckling causes a surge in maternal prolactin, which inhibits ovulation.
When ovulation occurs and fertilization occurs, "the contraceptive effect of breastfeeding
may be partly due to inhibiting implantation of a fertilized egg." [Kennedy K.I. in
Contraceptive Technology 18th Edition p. 578]

COST: None

ADVANTAGES OF BREASTFEEDING

Menstrual: Involution of the uterus occurs more rapidly; suppresses menses
Sexual/psychological: Breast-feeding pleasurable to many women
- Facilitates bonding between mother and child (if not stressful)

Cancers, tumors, and masses: Reduces risk of ovarian cancer and endometrial cancer;
possible slight protective effect against breast cancer if practiced long-term
Other:
- Provides the healthiest most "natural" food for baby
- Protects baby against asthma, allergies, URIs and diarrhea by passage of mother's
  antibodies into breastmilk
- Facilitates postpartum weight loss
- Less expensive and less time preparing bottles and feedings

DISADVANTAGES

Menstrual: Return to menses unpredictable

Sexual/psychological:

- Breastfeeding mother may be self-conscious in public or during intercourse
- Hypoestrogenism of breastfeeding may cause dyspareunia due to lack of lubrication
- Tender breasts may decrease sexual pleasure

Cancers, tumors, and masses: None

Other:

- Working women need to find time/place/resources to pump
- Effectiveness after 6 months is markedly reduced; return to fertility often precedes menses
- Frequent breastfeeding may be inconvenient or perceived as inconvenient
- No protection against STIs, HIV, AIDS
- If the mother is HIV+, there is a 14%-29% chance that HIV will be passed to infant via breast milk. Antiretroviral therapy decreases risk of transmission. Breastfeeding is not recommended for HIV+ women in the U.S.
- Sore nipples and breasts; risk of mastitis associated with breast-feeding

COMPLICATIONS: Risk of mastitis increases; return of fertility can precede menses

CANDIDATES FOR USE

- Amenorrheic women less than 6 months postpartum who exclusively breast-feed their babies
- Women free of a blood borne infection which could be passed to the newborn
- Women not on drugs which can adversely affect their babies

MEDICAL ELIGIBILITY CHECKLIST

Ask the patient the questions below. If she answers "NO" to ALL questions, she can use LAM. If she answers Yes to any questions, follow the instructions. Sometimes there is a way to incorporate LAM into her contraceptive plans; in other situations, LAM is contraindicated.

1. Is your baby 6 months old or older?

☐ No   ☐ Yes   Help her choose another method to supplement the contraceptive effect of LAM

2. Has your menstrual period returned? (Bleeding in the first 8 weeks after childbirth does not count)

☐ No   ☐ Yes   After 8 weeks postpartum, if a woman has 2 straight days of menstrual bleeding, or her menstrual period has returned, she can no longer count on LAM as her contraceptive. Help her choose method appropriate for breastfeeding woman

3. Have you begun to breastfeed less often? Do you regularly give the baby other food or liquid (other than water)?

☐ No   ☐ Yes   If the baby's feeding pattern has just changed, explain that patient must be fully or nearly fully breastfeeding around the clock to protect against pregnancy. If not, she cannot use LAM effectively. Help her choose method appropriate for breastfeeding woman

4. Has a health-care provider told you not to breastfeed your baby?

☐ No   ☐ Yes   If a patient is not breastfeeding, she cannot use LAM. Help her choose another method. A woman should not breastfeed if she is taking mood altering recreational drugs, reserpine, ergotamine, antimetabolites, cyclosporine, bromocriptine, tetracycline, radio-active drugs, lithium, or certain anticoagulants (heparin and coumadin are safe); if her baby has a specific infant metabolic disorder; or possibly if she carries viral hepatitis or is HIV positive.

All others can and should consider breastfeeding for the health benefits to the infant. In 1997, the FDA advised the manufacturer of Prozac (fluoxetine) to revise its labeling; it now states that "nursing while on Prozac is not recommended." On the other hand, Briggs notes that "the authors of a 1996 review stated that they encouraged women to continue breastfeeding while taking the drug" *[Nulman Tetralogy, 1996][Briggs, 2002]* This was also the conclusion of a 1999 review of the benefits of SSRIs for depressed breastfeeding women *[Edwards, 1999]*

5. Are you infected with HIV, the virus that causes AIDS?

☐ No ☐ Yes Where other infectious diseases kill many babies, mothers should be encouraged to breastfeed. HIV, however, may be passed to the baby in breast milk. When infectious diseases are a low risk and there is safe, affordable food for the baby, advise her to feed her baby that other food. Help her choose a birth control method other than LAM. A meta-analysis of published prospective trials estimated the risk of transmission of HIV with breastfeeding is 14% if the mother was infected prenatally but is 29% if the woman has her primary infection in the postpartum period

6. Do you know how long you plan to breastfeed your baby before you start supplementing his/her diet?

☐ No ☐ Yes In the U.S. the median duration of breastfeeding is approximately 3 months. Often breastfeeding women do not know when their menses will return, when they will start supplementing breastfeeding with other foods or exactly when they will stop breastfeeding their infant. It is wise to provide a woman with the contraceptive she will use when the answer to one of the above questions becomes positive and with a backup contraceptive and EC even during the period when breast-feeding is effective

INITIATING METHOD

- Patient should start exclusively breastfeeding immediately or as soon as possible after delivery
- Ensure that woman is breastfeeding fully or almost fully (>90% of baby's feedings); feedings around the clock
- A woman working outside of the home requires a breastfeeding-friendly environment, and preferably on-site childcare so that woman can visit her child every few hours to breastfeed; otherwise, breast pumping is needed
- Encourage use of second method of contraception if any questions about LAM effectiveness

INSTRUCTIONS FOR PATIENT

- Refer to lactation consultant/La Leche League for support/resources
  (www.lalecheleague.org)
- Breastfeed consistently, exclusively and correctly for maximum effectiveness
- Breast milk should constitute at least 90% of baby's feedings
- Think about methods that can be used once menses return or at 6 months

PROBLEM MANAGEMENT

Deficient milk supply:
- The more a breast is emptied, the more it fills up
- Commonly caused by insufficient nursing, use of artificial nipple (e.g. pacifier), fatigue or maternal stress
- Encourage woman to breastfeed often (8-10 times daily), eat well, get additional rest, drink lots of fluids and take prenatal vitamins and iron supplements

- Immediately postpartum women should breastfeed every 2-3 hours to stimulate milk production
- Seek assistance from a board certified lactation specialist
- Avoid estrogen-containing contraceptives

Sore nipples:
- Provide good support of breasts and psyche (inform her about La Leche League and of other lactation specialists)
- Commonly caused by incorrect application of the baby's mouth to the breast. Uncommonly caused by infection
- Check for correct ways of latching and suckling; be sure to break the suction before removing the baby from the breast
- Improve with practice; change the pressure points on the nipple by changing the baby's position for feeding
- Allow nipples to air dry with breast milk on the areola to reduce infection and nipple soreness. Apply lanolin to nipples after each feeding to decrease soreness after nipples have air dried
- Do not cleanse breasts other than with water at any time
- Cool gel packs are available to decrease soreness

Sore breasts:
- Wear a well-fitted, supportive nursing bra; avoid bras that are too tight or have underwire
- Apply heat on sore areas; some women apply teabag as compress on sore nipples
- Nurse frequently or use pump to get excess milk out of affected breast
- Encourage additional rest
- Seek medical evaluation if any erythema, fever or other signs or symptoms of infection develop

Other:
- Stress, fear, lack of confidence, lack of strong motivation to succeed at breastfeeding, lack of partner and/or societal support, and/or poor nutrition can cause problems

FERTILITY AFTER USE
Patient's baseline fertility (ability to become pregnant) is not altered once patient discontinues breastfeeding

TEN STEPS TO SUCCESSFUL BREASTFEEDING

From: Protecting, Promoting and Supporting Breastfeeding: The special role of maternity services. (A joint WHO/UNICEF statement. Geneva, World Health Organization, 1989)

All healthcare facilities where childbirth is undertaken should:

1. Have a written breastfeeding policy that is routinely communicated to all health care staff.
2. Train all health care staff in skills necessary to implement this policy.
3. Inform all pregnant women about the benefits and management of breastfeeding.
4. Help mothers initiate breastfeeding within the first 30 minutes after birth.
5. Show mothers how to breastfeed and how to maintain lactation even if they are separated from their infants because of a medical reason.
6. Give newborn infants no milk feeds or water other than breast milk unless indicated for a medical reason.
7. Allow mothers and infants to remain together 24 hours a day from birth.
8. Encourage natural breastfeeding on demand.
9. Do not give or encourage the use of artificial teats to breastfeed infants.
10. Promote the establishment of breastfeeding support groups and refer mothers to these on discharge from the hospital or clinic.

The importance of breastfeeding has been highlighted. Year 2010 goals: 75% of women will initiate breastfeeding and 50% will continue for 6 months

All breastfeeding women should be provided contraception because:
- Duration of breastfeeding in the U.S. is brief (median: under 3 months)
- Most couples resume intercourse a few weeks after delivery
- Ovulation may precede first menses

Table 16.1 *When to initiate contraception in breastfeeding women:*

METHOD	WHEN TO START IN LACTATING WOMEN	EFFECT ON BREAST MILK
Condoms (Male & Female), Sponge	• Immediately	No effect
Cervical Cap, Diaphragm	• 4-6 weeks postpartum, after cervix and vagina normalized (need to be refitted for postpartum women)	No effect
Progestin-Only Methods • Depo-Provera • Progestin – Only Pills • Implanon	• Most authorities, including National Medical Committee of the Planned Parenthood Federation of America, consider it appropriate to initiate any progestin-only method immediately postpartum • WHO and International Planned Parenthood Federation recommend waiting 6 weeks postpartum because of theoretical concerns for the newborn infant	• No significant impact on milk quality or production • Breast-feeding prolonged • Breast fed children of DMPA users grow at normal rate
Combined Pills or Combined Injections Patch Vaginal Ring	• American Academy of Pediatrics recommends use of low-dose combined hormonal contraceptives when infant' is not relying solely on breastmilk. No sooner than 3-6 weeks postpartum • Also, see Table 26.2 on pg. 105	Quality and quantity of breast milk may be diminished if used prior to establishment of lactation. After lactation establishment, low-dose COCs have no significant impact
IUD: • Copper • Levonorgestrel	• Usually await uterine involution to insert (4-6 weeks) • May insert Copper or LNG IUD within first 20 minutes after delivery of placenta with special equipment	No effect with Copper IUD; theoretical effect only; no demonstrated effect for Mirena
Tubal Sterilization	Usually done in first 24-48 hours postpartum, or await complete uterine involution for interval tubal sterilization (> 6 weeks postpartum)	No effect

CHAPTER 17
Fertility Awareness Methods (FAM)

www.dml.georgetown.edu/depts/irh OR www.usc.edu/hsc/info/newman/resource/nfp.html
www.cyclebeads.com OR www.irh.org

DESCRIPTION: A woman cannot identify the exact day of ovulation using FAM methods; rather she identifies when the fertile phase of her cycle begins and ends. A woman's fertile phase may begin 3-6 days before ovulation (because sperm can live in cervical mucus for ◄ 3-6 days); a woman's fertile phase ends 24 hours after ovulation

For purposes of FAM, a woman's menstrual cycle has 3 phases:

1. Infertile phase: before ovulation
2. Fertile phase: Approximately 5-7 days in the mid-portion of the cycle, including several days before and the day before and after ovulation;
3. Infertile phase: after ovulation

During the fertile phase, a couple should be abstinent to avoid pregnancy (periodic abstinence). Of the FAM methods discussed, the Calendar Method, Standard Days Method, and the Cervical Mucus Method can be used to identify the beginning and the end of the fertile period; the BBT Method can only be used to identify the end of the fertile period. Thus, couples using the BBT Method could only safely have unprotected intercourse during the post-ovulatory period, as the method cannot be used to define the pre-ovulatory infertile phase. As couples using either the Calendar or the Cervical Mucus Methods can theoretically identify the beginning and the end of the fertile period, they may have unprotected intercourse during the pre-ovulatory infertile phase and the post-ovulatory infertile phase. However, in order to minimize the chance of an unintended pregnancy, some advocate that couples only have unprotected intercourse during the post-ovulatory infertile phase regardless of the method of FAM they are using.

Techniques used to determine high-risk fertile days include:

1. Calendar Method: To calculate the fertile days:
   - Record days of menses prospectively for 6-12 cycles
   - Most estimates assume that sperm can survive 2-3 days and ovulation occurs 14 days before menses (motile sperm have been found as long as 7 days after intercourse and the extreme interval following a single act of coitus leading to an achieved pregnancy is 6 days *[Spcroff-1999]*)
   - Earliest day of fertile period = day # in a cycle corresponding to **shortest cycle length minus 18**
   - Latest day of fertile period = day # in a cycle corresponding to **longest cycle length minus 11**

2. Standard Days Method Utilizing Color-Coded Beads
   - For women with MOST cycles 26-32 days long, avoid UNPROTECTED intercourse on days 8-19 (white beads on CycleBead necklace). No need for 3-6 months of extensive cycle calculations
   - 4.75% failure over 1 year with perfect use; 11.96% with typical use *[Arevalo-2002]*
   - Resources available from the Institute for Reproductive Health, www.irh.org (CD, training manual, patient brochure, sample beads). Beads can also be ordered from www.cyclebeads.com

3. Cervical Mucus Ovulation Detection Method
   - Women check quantity and character of mucus on the vulva or introitus with fingers or tissue paper each day for several months to learn cycle:
     - Post-menstrual mucus: scant or undetectable
     - Pre-ovulation mucus: cloudy, yellow or white, sticky
     - Ovulation mucus: clear, wet stretches, sticky (but slippery)
     - Post-ovulation fertile mucus: thick, cloudy
     - Post-ovulation post-fertile mucus: scant or undetectable
   - When using method during preovulatory period, must abstain 24 hours after intercourse to make test interpretable as semen and vaginal fluids can obscure character of cervical mucus

- Abstinence or barrier method through fertile period (ie abstinence for a given cycle begins as soon as the woman notices any cervical secretions)
- Intercourse without restriction beginning 4th day after the last day of wet, clear, slippery mucus (post ovulation)

4. Basal Body Temperature Method (BBT)

- Assumes early morning temperature measured before arising will increase noticeably (0.4-0.8⁰ F) with ovulation; fertile period is defined as the day of first temperature drop or first elevation through 3 contive days of elevated temperature. Temperature drop does NOT always occur

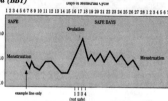

Figure 17.1 Basal body temperature variations during a menstrual cycle

- Abstinence begins first day of mentrual bleeding and lasts through 3 consecutive days of sustained temperature rise (at least 0.2⁰ C or 0.4⁰ F)

5. Post-ovulation Method

- Permits unprotected intercourse only after signs of ovulation (BBT, cervical mucus, etc) have subsided

6. Symptothermal Method

- Combines at least two methods — usually cervical mucus changes with BBT
- May also include mittelschmerz, change in libido, and changes in cervical texture, position and dilation to detect ovulation:
  - During preovulatory and ovulatory periods, cervix softens, opens and is moister
  - During postovulatory period, cervix drops, becomes firm and closes

EFFECTIVENESS (see Table 13.2, page 38)

NFP/FAM First-year failure rate (100 women-years of use)

Method	Typical use*	Perfect use
Calendar	25	9
Standard Days Method	12	5
Ovulation Method	25	3
Symptothermal	25	2
Post-ovulation	25	1

*FAM usually more effective than NFP [Trussell IN Contraceptive Technology, 2004]

MECHANISM: Abstinence or barriers during fertile period

COST: Training, supplies (special digital basal body thermometer, Cycle Beads, charts)

ADVANTAGES

Menstrual: No change. Helps woman learn more about her menstrual physiology
Sexual/psychological: Men and women can work together in using this method. Men must be aware that abstinence or use of second method is essential during the fertile period
Other:
- May be only method acceptable to couples for cultural or religious reasons
- Helps couples achieve pregnancy when practiced in reverse

DISADVANTAGES

Menstrual:
- Difficult to use in early adolescence, when approaching menopause, and in postpartum women when cycles are irregular (or absent)
- Even women with "regular" periods can vary as much as ± 7 days in any given cycle
- Cervical mucus techniques may be complicated by vaginal infections

Sexual/psychological:
- Requires abstinence, barrier method, or another contraceptive that does not change pattern of ovulation during 6-12 month learning/data-gathering period unless (CycleBead method is used)
- Complete abstinence in an anovulatory cycle, if using post-ovulation techniques. This method demands great self-control: either abstinence or use of another method must be used during long periods of time when woman is or may become fertile
- Requires rigorous discipline, good communication and full commitment of both partners
- Requires abstinence at time of ovulation, which is the time of peak libido

Cancers, tumors, and masses: None

Other:
- May not be helpful during time of stress
- Method very unforgiving of improper use
- Does not protect against STIs
- Relatively high failure rate with typical use
- Less reliable in settings of fever, vaginal infections, douching, and use of certain medications

COMPLICATIONS: None

CANDIDATES FOR USE

- Women with regular menstrual cycles at minimal risk for STIs
- Those with religious/cultural proscriptions against using other methods
- Highly motivated couples willing to commit to extensive abstinence or to use barriers during vulnerable periods

Adolescents: Not appropriate until regular menstrual cycles established

MEDICAL ELIGIBILITY CHECKLIST: Ask the woman the questions below. If she answers NO to ALL questions, she CAN use any fertility awareness-based method if she wants. If she answers YES to any question, follow the instructions. No conditions restrict use of these methods, but some conditions can make them harder to use effectively

1. Do you have a medical condition that would make pregnancy especially dangerous?

☐ No ☐ Yes She may want to choose a more effective method. If not, stress careful use of fertility awareness-based methods to avoid pregnancy and availability of EC

2. Do you have irregular or prolonged menstrual cycles? Vaginal bleeding between periods?
For younger women: Are your periods just starting?
For older women: Have your periods become irregular?

☐ No ☐ Yes Predicting her fertile time with only the calendar method may be hard or impossible. She can use basal body temperature (BBT) and/or cervical mucus, or she may prefer different method

3. Did you recently give birth or have an abortion? Are you breastfeeding? Do you have any other condition that affects menstrual bleeding?

☐ No   ☐ Yes   These conditions may affect fertility signs, making fertility awareness-based methods hard to use. For this reason, a woman or couple may prefer a different method. If not, they may need more counseling and follow-up to use the method effectively

4. If you recently stopped using Depo-Provera or combined hormonal methods, are your periods still irregular?

☐ No   ☐ Yes   If her cycles have not been re-established, she may need to use another method until cycles are regular

5. Do you have any infections or diseases that may change cervical mucus, basal body temperatures, or menstrual bleeding—such as sexually transmitted disease (STD) or pelvic inflammatory disease (PID) in the last 3 months, or vaginal infection?

☐ No   ☐ Yes   These conditions may affect fertility signs, making fertility awareness-based methods hard to use. Once an infection is treated and reinfection is avoided, however, a woman can use fertility awareness-based methods

INITIATING METHOD

- Requires several months of data collection and analysis unless using CycleBeads
- Description of methods
- Formal training necessary. Couples may be trained together
- Resources are available from:
  1. Calgary Billings Centre of Natural Family Planning, Room 1, 1247 Bel-Aire Dr SW, Calgary, AB T2V 2C1, (403) 252-3929, www.billings-centre.ab.ca
  2. California Association of Natural Family Planning, 1010 - 11th St, Suite 200, Sacramento, CA 95814, (877) 332-2637, www.canfp.org
  3. The Couple to Couple League International, PO Box 111184, Cincinnati, OH 45211-1184, (513) 471-2000, www.ccli.org
  4. Institute for Reproductive Health, Georgetown University, 4301 Connecticut Ave, NW, Suite 310, Washington, D.C. 20008, (202) 687-1392, www.irh.org
  5. National Center for Women's Health, Pope Paul VI Institute, 6901 Mercy Road, Omaha, NE 68106-2604, (402) 390-6600, www.popepaulvi.com
  6. Family of the Americas Foundation, Inc., PO Box 1170, Dunkirk, MD 20754-1170, (800) 443-3395, www.familyplanning.net
  7. Northwest Family Services, 4805 NE Glisan St, Portland, OR 97213, (503) 230-6377, www.nwfs.org
  8. Twin Cities NFP Center, HealthEast, St. Joseph's Hospital, 69 W Exchange St, St. Paul, MN 55102, (651) 232-3088, www.tcnfp.org

BUYER BEWARE   A woman considering use of the fertility awareness methods must be aware of several potential pitfalls, summarized in **the five "R's"**:

- **R**estrictions on sexual spontaneity (method requires extensive abstinence or the use of backup method)
- **R**igorous daily monitoring
- **R**equired training
- **R**isk of pregnancy during prolonged training period
- **R**isk of pregnancy high on unsafe days

INSTRUCTIONS FOR PATIENT

- Requires discipline, communication, listening skills, full commitment of both partners. Mistakes using this method are particularly likely to lead to unintended pregnancies as intercourse is then occurring at the time in the cycle when a woman *most* likely to become pregnant
- If using FAM, use contraception during fertile days
- If using NFP, abstain from sexual intercourse during fertile days
- Encourage other forms of sexual satisfaction

FOLLOW-UP

- Have you had sexual intercourse during "unsafe" times during your cycle?
- Discuss use of emergency contraception if having sex during "unsafe" times during cycle
- Do you have emergency contraceptive pills in your medicine chest? ⬅

PROBLEM MANAGEMENT

Inconsistent use and risk taking: Educate about emergency contraception when women start using method

FERTILITY AFTER DISCONTINUATION OF METHOD: No effect

The New TwoDay Method of Family Planning

The TwoDay method of familiy planning is based on identifying the fertile days of a woman's menstrual cycle. This method is grounded in research completed on the relationship of fertility signs to actual fertility as well as work that more precisely delineates the fertile days of the woman's menstrual cycle. *[Higers-1978]*

A good indicator of fertility is the change in cervical secretions during the menstrual cycle. The TwoDay method requires only that a woman monitor the presence or absence of secretions to determine on each day if she is fertile. She is taught to consider as 'secretions' anything that she perceives coming from her vagina, except menstrual bleeding. The woman then asks herself two simple questions: *(1) Did I note secretions today? (2) Did I note secretions yesterday?* If she notices any secretions (today or yesterday), she is probably fertile, and needs to abstain from unprotected intercourse if she wishes to avoid pregnancy. If she notices no secretions on both days, she is not fertile.

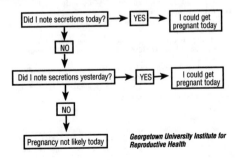

Georgetown University Institute for Reproductive Health

CHAPTER 18

Condoms for Men

DESCRIPTION

Condoms for men are sheaths made of latex, polyurethane or natural membranes (usually lamb cecum), which are placed over the penis prior to contact and worn until after ejaculation when the penis is removed from the orifice (vagina, mouth, anus). Latex condoms are available in at least 2 sizes, in a wide variety of textures and thicknesses (0.03-0.09 mm), and come with or without spermicidal coating. Two brands of polyurethane condoms are currently available in the US. When used correctly and consistently, male latex condoms are highly effective in preventing sexual transmission of HIV and can reduce the risk for other STDs (ie gonorrhea, chlamydia and trichomonas). Natural membrane condoms (made from the intestinal caecum of lambs) may not provide the same level of STI protection. Condoms may be used as a primary contraceptive method, as a back up method, or with another method to provide STI risk reduction. **When used as a primary contraceptive method, it is important that condoms be coupled with advance provision/prescription of emergency contraceptive pills (ECPs) since couples experience a condom break or slippage during approximately 3-5% of acts of intercourse:**

> If 14,000 acts of intercourse are protected by condoms, a mishap (breakage, slippage part of the way down the shaft of the penis, or slippage completely off the penis) will occur approximately 5% of the time or 700 times. If couples experiencing breakage or slippage identify this and use a single tablet of Plan B (0.75 mg levonorgestrel) within one hour, only one of those 700 women will experience an unintended pregnancy. The failure rate of a single tablet of Plan B within one hour of unprotected sex is 0.14% or just about 1 in 700 [Shelton - 2002]. Taking 2 tablets of Plan B is still recommended though to maximize efficacy.

EFFECTIVENESS [Trussell J IN Contraceptive Technology, 2004]

Perfect use failure rate in the first year of use: 2% (See Table 13.2, page 38)

If each couple had intercourse at the average coital frequency of 83 acts of intercourse per woman per year in the United States [Trussell-1995], then 100 couples would have had intercourse a combined total of 8,300 times over the course of a year. One pregnancy per 4,150 acts of intercourse is a remarkably low pregnancy rate (0.02%) [Warner-2004]

Typical use failure rate in the first year of use: 15%

- The most common reason for condom failure is not using a condom with every act of intercourse [Werner-2004] [Steiner-1999]
- Comparative testing has shown that latex and polyurethane condoms provide the same pregnancy protection. Polyurethane condoms are more likely to slip or break (8-10%) than latex condoms (1.6-1.7%)
- Dual use of a condom plus another contraceptive may dramatically reduce the risk of both pregnancy and STI. [Warner-2004][Cates-2002]. However, there is no evidence that spermicidal condoms are more effective than condoms without spermicide despite their higher cost and shorter shelf-life [Warner-2004][CDC-1998]

MECHANISM

- Condoms act as a barrier; they prevent the passage of sperm into the vagina. Sheathing the penis also reduces transmission and acquisition of STIs, including HIV. **Spermicidal condoms are no longer recommended at all as they provide no additional protection against pregnancy or STIs!** Most condom manufacturers have stopped producing ←— spermicidal condoms

COST

- Average retail cost for latex condoms is $0.50, but some designer condoms cost several dollars. Polyurethane condoms cost $.80-$2.00 each
- Public health agencies often offer free condoms. Purchasers of large numbers of condoms may buy condoms for as low as 4 to 6 cents per condom from Ansell and Durex

ADVANTAGES

Menstrual: No direct impact on menses, but couple may feel more comfortable

Sexual/psychological:

- Some men may maintain erection longer with condoms, making sex more enjoyable
- If the woman/partner puts the condom on, it may add to sexual pleasure
- Male involvement is encouraged and is essential!
- Availability of wide selection of condom types and designs can add variety
- Makes sex less messy for the woman by catching the ejaculate
- Intercourse may be more pleasurable because fear of pregnancy and STIs is decreased

Cancers/tumors & masses: Decrease in HIV transmission reduces risks of AIDS-related malignancies

Other:

- Consistent condom use reduces risks of HIV transmission by approximately 10-fold [Davis-1999] [Pinkerton-1997] [Warner-2004] See Figure 18.2, page 62
- Readily available over the counter; no medical visit required
- Usually inexpensive for single use
- Easily transportable. Don't leave in wallet too long; probably ok for 1 month. It has been suggested that a condom be placed between photographs in a wallet to protect against damage
- Opportunity for couples to improve communication and negotiating skills
- Immediately active after placement
- May reduce risk of PID, infertility, ectopic pregnancy and chronic pelvic pain

DISADVANTAGES: May break or fall off. *Options: see Fig. 18.3, p. 62*

Menstrual: None

Sexual/psychological:

- Use may interrupt lovemaking. Requires discipline to resist impulse to progress to intercourse after erection
- May cause man to lose erection
- Blunting of sensation or "unnatural" feeling with intercourse
- Plain condoms may decrease lubrication and provide less stimulation for woman (use water-based or silicone lubricant with latex condoms if this is a problem)
- Requires prompt withdrawal after ejaculation, which may decrease pleasure (especially the woman's pleasure)
- Makes sex messier for the man (getting rid of condom)

Cancers/tumors and masses: None

Other:

- Requires education/experience for successful use
- Either member of couple may have latex allergy or reaction to spermicide; polyurethane condom is appropriate alternative
- Users must avoid petroleum-based vaginal products when using latex condoms (Figure 18.1, p. 61). Polyurethane condom is appropriate alternative
- Couples may be embarrassed to purchase or to apply condoms due to taboos about touching genitalia, stigma of concern about STDs/HIV

COMPLICATIONS

- Allergic reactions to latex are rarely life threatening; 2-3% of Americans (men and women) have a latex allergy; up to 14% of individuals working with latex are latex sensitive. Polyurethane condoms do not cause allergic reactions
- Condom retained in vagina (uncommon) exposes woman to risk of infection as well as pregnancy. If this occurs: 1) try to remove by pinching with second and third fingers or 2) enlist partner's help or 3) go to clinician ASAP. Use EC ASAP

PRECAUTIONS

- Men who are unable to maintain erection when they wear condoms; benzocaine condoms by Durex are now available. Benzocaine is to prevent premature ejaculation
- Men with abnormal ejaculatory pathways not sheathed by condom
- Woman whose partners will not use condoms
- Women who require high contraceptive efficacy should, at a minimum, add another method in addition to the condom
- Couples in which either partner has latex allergy should avoid latex condoms; men can use Durex-Avanti or Trojan-Supra; women can use Reality female condom
- Couples in which either partner has spermicide allergy or is at high risk for HIV should avoid spermicide-coated condoms

CANDIDATES FOR USE

- Anyone at risk for an STI; appropriate for most couples
- May be used alone or coupled with a second contraceptive method

Special applications for infection control:
- Non-monogamous couples (i.e. if either partner has multiple partners)
- During pregnancy as well as at all other times
- After delivery or pregnancy loss to reduce risk of endometritis (although abstinence is preferable)
- Couples with known viral infections (HIV, HPV, HSV-2) in areas completely covered by device

Adolescents: Excellent option, especially when combined with another method

INITIATING METHOD

Couples desiring to use condoms often benefit from concrete instructions. Use a model and actual condom. Counsel new users about:
- Options among condom types
- Storage for safety and ready access
- How to negotiate condom use with partner and when to place condom [Warner-2004]
- How to open package and place correct side of condom over penis
- How to unroll and allow space for ejaculate (depending on condom design)

Provide ECPs to couples relying on the condom for birth control to insure immediate use in the event of condom mishap or problem. This will minimize risk of unintended pregnancy

INSTRUCTIONS FOR PATIENTS (See Figure 18.1, pg. 61)

- Learn how to use a condom long before you need it. Both women and men need to know how. Practice with models: fingers or man's penis
- Buy condoms in advance, carry with you; Keep extra condoms out of sunlight and heat
- Try new condoms to find favorite size, scent, and texture and to add variety
- Check date on condom carefully. It may be an expiration date OR a date of production. If it is an expiration date, do not use beyond expiration date. If it is a date of production, condom may be used for several years from the date of production (2 years for spermicidal condoms, 5 years for nonspermicidal latex condoms)

- Open package carefully, squeeze condom out, avoid tearing with fingernails, teeth, etc.
- Use appropriate water-based or silicon-based lubricant with latex condoms (see page 61). Never put lubricant inside the condom

Researchers at Univ. Texas Galveston found 3 vaginal lubricants that are safe, non-irritating (unlike Nonoxynol-9) and strongly inhibited HIV replication in vitro: Astroglide, Vagisil and ViAmor. [AIDS Research and Human Retroviruses-2001].

- Place condom over penis before any genital contact. Either partner can put it on!
- Consider placing a second condom (larger size) over lubricated condom if history of previous breakage or if man has any evidence of STI
- If condom used for oral or rectal intercourse replace with a new condom prior to vaginal entry
- Vigorous sex can break the condom. Consider using 2 condoms at once
- Immediately after ejaculation (before loss of erection) hold rim of condom against shaft of penis and remove condom-covered penis from vagina (or anus). One study found only 71% of men held the rim of the condom during withdrawal and only 50% withdrew immediately after ejaculation [Warner-1999]
- Remove condom from the penis and inspect carefully for any breaks
- Dispose of used condom. Do not reuse
- If a condom falls off, slips, tears or breaks, start using ECPs as soon as possible. If you do not have ECPs, call 1-888-NOT-2-LATE or check www.not-2-late.com to find out how to get them. In some states, you can get EC from a pharmacist without a prescription. If any risk for STIs, seek medical care

FOLLOW-UP
- Are you and your partner comfortable using condoms?
- Have you had any problems with using the condom? Breaking? Slipping off? Decreased sensation? Vaginal soreness with use? Skin irritation or redness during the day after using it?
- Have you had any post-coital "yeast infection" symptoms? (A woman may confuse an allergic reaction to the condom and/or spermicide with a candidal infection)
- Have you had intercourse—even once—without a condom?
- Did you have any questions about ECPs? ◄
- Do you have Plan B ECPs in your medicine chest? ◄
- Do you plan to have children? OR Do you plan to have more children? When?

PROBLEM MANAGEMENT
Allergic reaction: [See Warner-2004]
- Beware that latex powder can induce anaphylaxis and that the severity of allergic reaction increases with continued exposure. Sometimes a person who says he (or she) is *"allergic"* to condoms may mean condoms are a) difficult to put on or b) lead to loss of erection or c) the couple simply doesn't like condoms or d) is being irritated by a spermicide or lubricant or e) an ongoing infection may be causing irritation. Irritation can also be caused by thrusting during sex. Couple may try another brand of latex condoms ◄
- Switch to polyurethane condoms (Durex, 2 Avanti Super or Trojan-Supra male condoms, Mayer Laboratories eZ-on, or Reality female condom) or stop using spermicide ◄ (depending on the suspected allergen or irritant)
- Switch to another approach to reducing STI risk and contraception, such as the female condom for STI risk reduction and a hormonal method for contraceptive effectiveness

Condom breakage: (Figure 18.3, p. 62) (1-2% for latex condoms)
- Insure correct technique. Common problems: pre-placement manipulations (stretching, etc), use of inappropriate lubricant (placement inside condom), and prolonged or extremely vigorous sex
- May need to recommend larger condom. The 16th edition of ***Contraceptive Technology*** (pages 147-152) lists characteristics of hundreds of U.S. condoms. The largest are: Kimono, Kimono Microthin, Magnum, MAXX, and Trojan Very Sensitive
- If couple using polyurethane, consider switching to latex condom
- May need to switch method
- Confirm that woman is using ECPs and has supply available at home

Condom slippage: (Figure 18.3, p. 62) (More common than condom breakage)
- Ensure correct technique. Common problems: condom not fully unrolled, lubricant placed incorrectly on inside of condom, and excessive delay in removing penis from vagina after ejaculation. Use of proper-sized condom is important (if condom is too large it may slip off)
- Rule out erectile dysfunction. Condoms may not be appropriate if man loses erection with condom placement or use
- Confirm that woman is using ECPs and has supply available at home

Decreased sensation:
- Common causes: condom too small, too thick or too tightly applied; inadequate lubrication
- Suggest experimentation with different textured condoms or placing second (larger size) condom over inner lubricated condom. Thinner condoms now available
- Integrate condom placement into lovemaking (suggest partner place condom to help arouse/excite man)

FERTILITY AFTER DISCONTINUATION OF METHOD
- Does not affect baseline fertility
- May protect fertility by reducing risk of STIs

To purchase the 18th edition of ***Contraceptive Technology***, with an excellent chapter on condoms by David Lee Warner (CDC) and Markus Steiner (FHI), call (706) 265-7435 or go to www.managingcontraception.com

Figure 18.1

HOW TO USE A LATEX CONDOM
(...Or rubber, sheath, prophylactic, safe, french letter, raincoat, glove, sock)

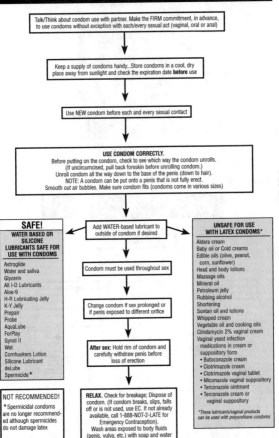

Talk/Think about condom use with partner. Make the FIRM commitment, in advance, to use condoms without exception with each/every sexual act (vaginal, oral or anal)

↓

Keep a supply of condoms handy...Store condoms in a cool, dry place away from sunlight and check the expiration date **before** use

↓

Use NEW condom before each and every sexual contact

↓

USE CONDOM CORRECTLY.
Before putting on the condom, check to see which way the condom unrolls.
(If uncircumcised, pull back foreskin before unrolling condom.)
Unroll condom all the way down to the base of the penis (down to hair).
NOTE: A condom can be put onto a penis that is not fully erect.
Smooth out air bubbles. Make sure condom fits (condoms come in various sizes)

↓

SAFE!
WATER BASED OR SILICONE LUBRICANTS SAFE FOR USE WITH CONDOMS

Astroglide
Water and saliva
Glycerin
All I-D Lubricants
Aloe-9
H-R Lubricating Jelly
K-Y Jelly
Prepair
Probe
AquaLube
ForPlay
Gynol II
Wet
Cornhuskers Lotion
Silicone Lubricant
deLube
Spermicide *

NOT RECOMMENDED!
* Spermicidal condoms are no longer recommended although spermicides do not damage latex

Add WATER-based lubricant to outside of condom if desired

↓

Condom must be used throughout sex

↓

Change condom if sex prolonged or if penis exposed to different orifice

↓

After sex: Hold rim of condom and carefully withdraw penis before loss of erection

↓

RELAX. Check for breakage; Dispose of condom. (If condom breaks, slips, falls off or is not used, use EC. If not already available, call 1-888-NOT-2-LATE for Emergency Contraception).
Wash areas exposed to body fluids (penis, vulva, etc.) with soap and water

UNSAFE FOR USE WITH LATEX CONDOMS*

Aldara cream
Baby oil or Cold creams
Edible oils (olive, peanut, corn, sunflower)
Head and body lotions
Massage oils
Mineral oil
Petroleum jelly
Rubbing alcohol
Shortening
Suntan oil and lotions
Whipped cream
Vegetable oil and cooking oils
Clindamycin 2% vaginal cream
Vaginal yeast infection medications in cream or suppository form
• Butoconazole cream
• Clotrimazole cream
• Clotrimazole vaginal tablet
• Miconazole vaginal suppository
• Terconazole ointment
• Terconazole cream or vaginal suppository

*These lubricants/vaginal products can be used with polyurethane condoms

Figure 18.2   10 Studies demonstrating protective effect of latex condoms against HIV transmission in heterosexual couples

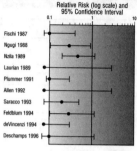

Relative Risk (log scale) and
95% Confidence Interval

Fischi 1987
Ngugi 1988
Nzila 1989
Laurian 1989
Plummer 1991
Allen 1992
Saracco 1993
Feldblum 1994
deVincenzi 1994
Deschamps 1996

[Feldblum et al., 1995]

Figure 18.3

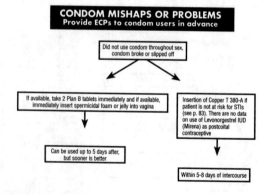

CONDOM MISHAPS OR PROBLEMS
Provide ECPs to condom users in advance

Did not use condom throughout sex, condom broke or slipped off

If available, take 2 Plan B tablets immediately and if available, immediately insert spermicidal foam or jelly into vagina

Can be used up to 5 days after, but sooner is better

Insertion of Copper T 380-A if patient is not at risk for STIs (see p. 83). There are no data on use of Levonorgestrel IUD (Mirena) as postcoital contraceptive

Within 5-8 days of intercourse

DESCRIPTION: The FC Female Condom (Formerly Reality) ◄

A condom inserted by women (or partner). Disposable, single-use **polyurethane** sheath, which is placed into the vagina. Flexible and movable inner ring at closed end is used to insert device into the vagina. Larger, fixed outer ring remains outside the vagina to cover part of introitus. Shelf life 3-5 years. When used as primary method, the female condom should be coupled with advance prescription of emergency contraceptive pills (ECPs)

EFFECTIVENESS *[Trussell J. IN Contraceptive Technology, 2004]*
Perfect use failure rate in first year of use: 5% (Table 13.2, pg. 38)
Typical use failure rate in first year of use: 21%

MECHANISM

- The female condom acts as a mechanical barrier; it prevents pregnancy by preventing the passage of sperm into the female reproductive tract
- Sheathing reduces transmission and acquisition of bacterial and viral STIs into the vagina and upper reproductive tract

COST in 2004: $3.30-$6.00 each; Price at public clinic: About $1.50 in 2004 ◄

ADVANTAGES

Menstrual: No impact on menses per se, but couple may feel more comfortable having intercourse during menses if a female condom is used. No data on risk of toxic shock syndrome

Sexual/psychology
- Intercourse may be more pleasurable because fear of pregnancy and STIs is decreased
- Can be inserted up to 8 hours before sex to allow more spontaneity
- If woman inserts it, she can be sure she is somewhat protected
- Makes sex less messy for the women after removal of the condom

Cancers/tumor, masses: no data

Other
- Available over-the-counter; no medical visit required
- Immediately active after placement
- Provides option to women whose partners can not or will not use male condom. May circumvent erectile concerns some men have with male condoms
- Although studies are lacking, is expected to reduce risk of fluid borne STI and HIV transmission and acquisition
- Can be safely used by people with latex allergies or sensitivities
- May possibly reuse for contraceptive purposes but NOT if being used to prevent infections. Reuse is generally not recommended. If women want to wash and reuse Reality condom, WHO recommendations are as follows:
  1) soak in bleach for 1 minute (kills HIV, HSV-2, CT, GC - 1 part bleach to 20 parts water) 2) Rinse with water 3) Wash gently with soap and water and pat dry 4) Store in clean, dry place. May reuse up to 5 times

DISADVANTAGES

Menstrual: None

Sexual/psychology:

- Use may interrupt lovemaking unless woman inserts beforehand in anticipation of intercourse
- Requires careful sexual practices during intercourse (see INSTRUCTIONS FOR PATIENT), which may make intercourse awkward and less spontaneous
- May be difficult for woman to ask her partner to follow instructions for use
- Noise made during intercourse may be distracting (additional lubricant can quiet)
- In one study, 88% of women and 91% of men disliked using the Reality Female Condom *[Duerr-Macaluso,-1999]*

Cancers/tumors/masses: None

Other:

- Somewhat difficult for new users (even experienced diaphragm users)
- Requires new condom with each act of intercourse
- Requires education and experience for successful use
- Couples may be embarrassed to purchase and to apply condoms due to taboos about touching genitalia; stigma of concern about STDs/HIV

COMPLICATIONS: Intravaginal methods can change vaginal flora and increase UTI risks

PRECAUTIONS

- Women unable to insert condom correctly and follow other instructions
- Women who require better pregnancy protection should at least combine the female condom with a more effective method (not the male latex condom)
- Stress not to wash and reuse a second or third time unless having sexual intercourse with same partner. New studies demonstrate that this condom may maintain its efficacy for several acts of intercourse. However, reuse is still generally <u>not</u> recommended, especially if using to prevent infection. No clinical studies available on the effectiveness after reuse.

CANDIDATES FOR USE: Except for women with pelvic relaxation, any woman may use the female condom. However, the female condom's relatively high cost, difficulty of use, and its high failure rate usually limit its use to women whose partners cannot or will not use a male condom. Specific candidates include:

- Couples willing to accept relatively high failure rates
- Couples who need method directed by woman
- Women needing protection postpartum (if intercourse not uncomfortable)

Special applications for infection control in couples not able to use male condoms:

- Non-monogamous couples (pregnant or not pregnant)
- New couples
- Before complete uterine involution, after pregnancy or after pregnancy loss, to reduce risk of endometritis
- Couples with known chronic viral infections (HIV, HPV, HSV) involved in areas sheathed by device

Adolescents: May be offered method, but cost, problems with proper placement and high failure rate detract from its desirability

INITIATING METHOD

- Women planning to use the female condom need to have a chance to study instructions and practice inserting and using method prior to relying on it; 25% in one study could not insert a female condom into their vagina even after having practiced inserting one into a plastic model *[Artz-2002]*
- Patients also benefit from counseling about:
  - How to negotiate with partner to be able to successfully use
  - Need to use with every act of intercourse and how to deal with device mishaps
- In addition, provide ECPs to women relying on female condoms for birth control to ensure immediate use after condom failures. This will minimize risk of unintended pregnancy

INSTRUCTIONS

- Open packaging carefully. Avoid scissors or sharp objects that could cut or tear device
- Patient should rest comfortably in squat or lithotomy position
- Compress inner ring of device and introduce into vagina much like a diaphragm. Use inner ring to guide sheath high into vagina until the outer ring rests against vulva. Rotate inner ring to stabilize device in vault. Avoid tearing condom with fingernails or jewelry. See package instructions for details and drawings illustrating insertion
- Penis should be manually placed (by either man or woman) into the sheath for intercourse and care should be taken to avoid penile contact outside the female condom
- Man should monitor for any friction between penis and device which can cause condom breakage or device inversion
- Remove condom immediately after intercourse. Test condom for patency and discard
- If there is any dislocation of the female condom during intercourse or any breakage or spillage of the ejaculate into genitalia, have patient start her ECPs ASAP. If woman has no ECPs, have her call 1-888-NOT-2-LATE or check www.not-2-late.com/ to locate a provider of ECPs in her area (available through pharmacist in some states). If at risk for STIs when condom fails, seek medical care
- CAUTION: When a latex male condom is used with a polyurethane female condom theoretically there can be an increased risk of breakage of either or both condoms.

FOLLOW-UP

- Have you had any problems using the female condom?
- Have you had intercourse—even once—without using a condom?
- Do you know how to use ECPs? Do you need more ECPs?
- Do you plan to have children? OR Do you plan to have more children? When?

PROBLEM MANAGEMENT

- Difficulty inserting device: Offer to formally (re)instruct patient
- Problems with removal: Recommend relaxation techniques or have partner remove
- Condom dislodgement or penis inserted outside condom: insert a new condom prior to continuing intercourse. Use ECPs if any spill suspected. If at risk for STIs, seek medical care

FERTILITY AFTER DISCONTINUATION OF METHOD

- Method has no effect on baseline fertility; immediate return of fertility
- Female condom may protect fertility by reducing risk of cervical or vaginal STIs, which can cause upper tract disease and subsequent infertility

CHAPTER 20
Cervical Caps
www.cervcap.com, www.femcap.com, www.lea.com,
www.plannedparenthood.org

DESCRIPTION

Three caps are now approved: Prentif, FemCap and Lea's Shield. Production of the Prentif Cavity Rim Cervical Cap has stopped. The company producing Prentif cervical caps has gone out of business. FemCap is silicone (latex-free) and is reuseable for up to 2 years. The Lea's Shield is latex-free. When used as a primary method, cervical caps should be coupled with advance prescription of emergency contraceptive pills (ECPs). Information about the Prentif cervical cap remains as many of these are in circulation. Chapter will be revised to focus more on Fem Cap and Lea's Shield in the next edition of ***Managing Contraception***

EFFECTIVENESS: The failure rate for FemCap in the package insert is 29%

MECHANISM

Acts both as a mechanical barrier to sperm migration into the cervical canal and as a chemical agent by applying the spermicide directly to the cervix

ADVANTAGES
Menstrual: None
Sexual/psychological
  • Intercourse may be more pleasurable because fear of pregnancy is reduced
  • Controlled by the woman
  • Can be inserted up to 6 hours prior to sexual intercourse to permit spontaneity in lovemaking
  • Can remain in place for multiple acts of sexual intercourse for up to 48 hours total from time of placement
Cancers, tumors, and masses: None
Other:
  • May reduce risk of cervical infections, including gonorrhea, chlamydia and PID, but should not be assumed to be protective against HIV infection as effective use requires use of a spermicide
  • Immediately active after placement
  • May be used during lactation

DISADVANTAGES
Menstrual: None
Sexual/psychological
  • Requires placement prior to genital contact, which may reduce spontaneity of sex
  • Some women do not like placing fingers or foreign body into vagina
Cancers, tumors, and masses
  • Labeling requires repeat Pap smear at 3 months after initiation because increased risk of cervical dysplasia at 3 months; no increase at 1 year. Data submitted to FDA in follow-up studies shows no increase in dysplasia
Other:
• Lack of protection against some STIs and HIV. Must use condoms if at risk
• Relatively high failure rate, especially in parous women
• Must be refitted postpartum or if large weight change since cervix changes

- Requires professional fitting and requires formal (although brief) training
- About 80% of women can be fitted
- Severe obesity or arthritis may make it difficult for patient to place correctly
- Odor may develop if cap left in place too long, if not appropriately cleansed, or if used during bacterial vaginosis

COMPLICATIONS
- UTIs may increase with Prentif Cavity Rim Cervical Cap (but not with FemCap)
- Cervical erosion may occur causing vaginal spotting and/or cervical discomfort. Some women change size of cervix during cycle and need two different size caps
- No cases of toxic shock have been reported, but theoretically, the risk may be increased, particularly if cap were left in for longer than recommended or used during menses
- Allergic reactions to latex may be life threatening

CANDIDATES FOR USE: Women NOT at risk for HIV
- Women willing and able to insert device prior to coitus and remove it later
- Women with smooth symmetrical cervix which can be fit successfully
- Women with pelvic relaxation are better candidates for cap than for diaphragm
- Women and partner(s) who have no allergies to spermicides

Adolescents: appropriate option, but fitting and insertion may be difficult and offers no protection against certain STIs including HIV. Requires high motivation level

INITIATING METHOD
- Given the high failure rates for the cervical cap, it is very important to provide ECPs in advance to enable immediate use after cervical cap dislodgement or non-use
- The cervical cap must be professionally fit and refit after each pregnancy
- A speculum exam is advisable, to evaluate for acute cervicitis and vaginitis, and to obtain a Pap smear
- If no nodules, lesions, cysts or other vaginal or cervical abnormalities preclude cap use, a rough estimate is made of the diameter of the cervix
- On bimanual exam, the uterine size and position, and the position, length and diameter of the cervix are determined
- Starting with the smallest likely size cap, squeeze the sides of the rim together and hold the cap with the dome pointing downward
- Apply a small amount of lubricant to the outside edge to facilitate insertion, but not on rim as that would interfere with vacuum creation
- With the patient in the lithotomy position, separate her labia and gently insert the cap into the vagina. Guide it into place until the rim slides over the sides of the cervix
- Check for adequate cervical coverage, proper seal and position stability
- The dome of the cap should completely cover the cervix; the rim of the cap tucked snugly and evenly into the fornices; there should be no gap between rim and cervix
- The cap should adhere to the cervix firmly; it should not dislodge during the fitting exam
- To evaluate the fit, make a 360° sweep of the cap rim with the vaginal examining finger to search for gaps or exposed parts of the cervix
- If a gap is found, see if the rim can be pulled away with direct pressure
- After the cap has been in place for at least a minute, check the suction by pinching the excess rubber on the dome between the tips of two fingers and tugging
- The dome should dimple but should not collapse
- Cap should not be dislodged by manual manipulations such as gently pushing and tugging on it with one or two fingers from several angles

- After successful fitting, remove the cap by pushing the rim away from the cervix with one or two fingers to break the suction and then gently pull the cap out of the vagina
- Have patient demonstrate her ability to insert and remove cervical cap

INSTRUCTIONS FOR PATIENT TO USE

- Fill the bottom 1/3 of the inner aspect of the cap with 2% spermicide jelly. Put the cap in
- Test the fit to insure cervix is covered, sweep with finger 360° around device and check that there are no gaps between the cervix and the cap. After suction develops for about 1 minute, check that the device does not dislodge with pressure
- Keep the cap in place for 6 hours after last sexual intercourse
- If multiple acts of sexual intercourse occur, there is no need to add more spermicide but do verify correct placement of the device before each episode of sexual intercourse
- Do not use the cap for more than 48 hours at a time, at the time of an infection, or during menses
- Do not expose the Prentif (latex) cap to petroleum-based products such as vaseline, baby oil, fungicidal creams and petroleum-based antibiotic creams (Listed in figure 18.1, p. 61)
- If cap dislodges, ECPs should be used ASAP. If woman has no ECPs, have her call 1-888-NOT-2-LATE or check www.not-2-late.com to locate a provider of ECPs in her area.
- Use a backup method for first few uses
- Combining the cervical cap and the male condom can increase pregnancy protection and decrease STD transmission
- The FDA recommends a follow-up Pap smear after 3 months
- Do not use cap for at least 2 or 3 days prior to Pap smears

HOW TO REMOVE

- Cap should not be removed until 6 hours after last ejaculation, but prior to 48 hours of use
- Insert a finger into the vagina until the rim of the cap is felt
- Press the cap rim until the seal against the cervix is broken; then tilt the cap off the cervix
- Hook finger around the rim and pull it sideways out of the vagina
- The device must be washed, rinsed, dried and stored in a cool, dark and dry location. Rinsing in Listerine can prevent odors. Corn starch may keep cap dry

FOLLOW-UP

- Are you or your partner experiencing any tenderness or irritation?
- Is the odor of the cap a problem?
- Do you use the cap every single time you have sexual intercourse?
- Do you have more ECPs in your medicine chest? ←
- Do you plan to have children? OR Do you plan to have more children? If yes, when?

PROBLEM MANAGEMENT

- Allergic reaction to latex: Stop use and switch to a non-latex method
- Spotting/cervical tenderness/erosion: Stop use to allow healing; refit with larger cap; rule out STI
- Malodor of device: Listerine soaks may help; shorten time left in place, or replace cap
- Failure to use correctly: Use emergency contraception. If not already available, call 1-888-NOT-2-LATE or check www.not-2-late.com

FERTILITY AFTER DISCONTINUATION OF METHOD: Immediate return to baseline fertility

DESCRIPTION: Latex rubber dome-shaped device filled with spermicide and placed to cover cervix; three types of diaphragms are available:

- Arcing spring: exerts pressure evenly around its rim to cover the cervix
- Coil spring: most appropriate for women with a deep pubic arch with average vaginal tone
- Wide spring: extends inward from the rim to contain the spermicide. Available only through manufacturer

EFFECTIVENESS (See Table 13.2, p. 39)

Perfect use failure rate in first year: 6%

Typical use failure rate in first year: 16%

[Trussell J IN Contraceptive Technology 2004]

Arcing Spring

MECHANISM

Acts both as a mechanical barrier to sperm migration into the cervical canal and as a spermicide

Coil Spring

ADVANTAGES

Menstrual: None

Wide Seal Rim

Sexual/psychological:

- Controlled by the woman
- May be placed by the woman in anticipation of intercourse (within 6 hrs)
- May make sexual intercourse more enjoyable by reducing risk of pregnancy

Cancers, tumors, and masses: None

Other:

- Reduces risk for cervical STIs, including gonorrhea, chlamydia, cervical dysplasia, and PID
- May be used during lactation after vagina and cervix have achieved non-pregnant shape
- Immediately active after placement

DISADVANTAGES: *"It's such a long way from the bed to the bathroom!"*

Menstrual: None

Sexual/psychological:

- Requires placement prior to genital contact which can interrupt spontaneity
- Taste of spermicide may discourage certain foreplay activities
- May become messy with multiple acts of intercourse
- Some women dislike placing fingers or foreign bodies into vagina

Cancer, tumors, and masses: None

Other:

- **Requires formal training and some dexterity to place and remove device**
- Requires professional fitting
- May not be feasible for women with pelvic relaxation
- May develop odor if not properly cleansed
- Severe obesity or arthritis may make insertion/removal difficult

COMPLICATIONS

- Increases risk of UTI, as result of pressure on urethra
- May increase risk of toxic shock syndrome, if used for prolonged periods during menses
- Large, poorly fitted diaphragm may cause vaginal erosions
- Allergic reaction to rubber

CANDIDATES FOR USE: Women NOT at risk for HIV

- Women who can predict when intercourse will occur! Important!
- Couples willing to interrupt sex to insert if not done beforehand
- Highly motivated women willing to use with every coital act
- Women able to insert and remove diaphragm
- Women with no allergy to latex

Adolescents: Appropriate, if taught to use consistently and correctly; requires discipline

INITIATING METHOD

- Given the high failure rates among users of the diaphragm it is extremely important that clinicians provide women ECPs in advance!
- Needs to be professionally fitted
- Examination with speculum will rule out any vaginal/cervical abnormalities
- On bimanual exam, determine degree of version of uterus; not a good method for extremely anteverted or retroverted cervix. Introduce your third finger into the posterior fornix and tilt your wrist upward to mark where on your index finger/hand contacts the symphysis. Use that measurement as a guide to select the size diaphragm to use and place a fitting diaphragm in the vagina
- Check to ensure diaphragm is lodged behind symphysis and completely covers the cervix. Have patient bear down and digitally check to ensure that diaphragm does not move from behind pubic arch
- Have woman walk around for a while in your office to test its long-term comfort
- Have woman demonstrate her ability to insert and remove diaphragm
- Encourage use of a backup method for first few uses to ensure correct use before relying exclusively on diaphragm for protection
- Suggest patient wear diaphragm for 6 hours before using it for contraception to ensure that it is comfortable and can be worn for 6 hours after intercourse

INSTRUCTIONS FOR USE

- Fill inner surface of device 2/3 full with 2 teaspoons of spermicide prior to insertion. It can remain in place for up to 24 hours total from time of placement. Place before genital contact but no longer than 6 hours before coitus

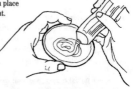

Figure 21.1 Risk of pregnancy increases when a spermicide is not used. Put spermicide on outside and on inside

- Prior to each act of coitus, reconfirm correct placement. For the second and each subsequent act, do not remove diaphragm but use a condom for additional protection. Current advice is that a spermicide NOT be used more than once each 24 hours.
- Leave in place for 6 hours after the last act of sexual intercourse
- Avoid using any petroleum-based vaginal products such as Vaseline, antifungal creams or some antibiotic creams. (See list of products UNSAFE to use with latex condoms on Figure 18.1, p. 61)
- After removal, clean with soap and water, rinse, dry, and store in the case in a cool, clean, dry, dark area. Corn starch may keep diaphragm dry
- Inspect periodically for any stiffness, holes, cracks, or other defects
- Have it checked each year by a professional. Replace at least every 2 years. Recheck for correct fit whenever there is a 20% weight change and after each pregnancy
- Combine diaphragm with male condoms to reduce pregnancy and STI risk
- If diaphragm dislodges or is not used properly, use EC

**Figure 21.2
Reconfirm correct placement of the diaphragm by feeling the cervix through the diaphragm**

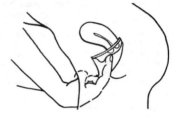

FOLLOW-UP
- Is the diaphragm comfortable? Do you feel excessive pressure?
- Do you get bladder infections often?
- Have you or your partner had an allergic reaction, i.e., burning or itching?
- Do you use the diaphragm consistently? If not, what keeps you from using this method everytime? Do you carry your diaphrapm with you if you will have intercourse away ← from home?
- Do you always apply a spermicide prior to insertion?
- Do you have ECPs in your medicine chest? ←
- Do you plan to have children? OR Do you plan to have more children? If yes, when?

PROBLEM MANAGEMENT
Prone to cystitis: Urinate postcoitally to reduce bladder colonization with vaginal bacteria; check fit to make sure there is not excessive urethral pressure
Allergy to latex: Discontinue use and discuss alternatives. Mylex makes a silicone diaphragm

FERTILITY AFTER DISCONTINUATION OF METHOD: No adverse effects on
fertility; may reduce risk of PID. Immediate return to baseline fertility

DESCRIPTION

The search for an effective vaginal microbicide that would also kill sperm remains an important research priority, perhaps the most important research priority, in reproductive health. In the USA, nonoxynol-9 (N-9) is available over the counter. In addition to N-9, patients around the world use menfegol, benzalkonium chloride, sodium docusate, and chlorhexidine (but these compounds are not available in the U.S.). Spermicides are available as vaginal creams, films, foams, gels, suppositories, sponges and tablets.

> Women at high risk of HIV should not use spermicides (WHO:4). Nor should women ◄ who are HIV-infected (WHO:4) *[WHO Medical Eligibility Guidelines-2004]* Condoms without nonoxynol-9 lubrication are effective and widely available. Women at high risk of HIV infection should also avoid using diaphragms and cervical caps to which nonoxynol-9 is added (WHO:3). The contraceptive effectiveness of diaphragms and cervical caps without nonoxynol-9 has been insufficiently studied and should be assumed to be less than that of diaphragms and cervical caps with nonoxynol-9.
>
> The Food and Drug Administration has proposed a labeling change for N-9 products that will indicate that these products may actually increase the possibility of acquiring HIV and other STDs from infected partners.

EFFECTIVENESS (See Trussell's failure rates, Table 13.2, p. 39)

Perfect use failure rate in first year: 15%

Typical use failure rate in first year: 29%   *[Trussell J IN Contraceptive Technology 2004]*

While an application of a spermicide into the vagina is an appropriate backup contraceptive (including use with a condom), **spermicidal condoms are no longer recommended at all** ◄ as they provide no additional protection against pregnancy or STIs. *[Warner-2004]*

MECHANISM

As barriers, the vehicles prevent sperm from entering the cervical os. As detergents, the chemicals attack the sperm flagella and body, reducing motility

ADVANTAGES

Menstrual: None

Sexual/psychological:
- Lubrication may heighten satisfaction for either partner
- Ease in application (for some women) prior to sexual intercourse
- Either partner can purchase and apply; requires minimal negotiation

Other:
- Available over the counter; requires no medical visit
- Inexpensive and easy to use
- Foam and spermicidal jelly are immediately active with placement
- May be used during lactation

DISADVANTAGES
Menstrual: None
Sexual/psychological:

- Films and suppository spermicides require 15 minutes for activation, which may interrupt or delay lovemaking
- Must feel comfortable inserting fingers into vagina
- Insertion is not easy for some couples due to embarrassment or reluctance to touch genitalia
- Some forms, e.g., foam, become "messy" during intercourse
- Possible vaginal, oral, and anal irritation can disrupt or preclude sex
- Taste may be unpleasant

Cancers, tumors, and masses: None
Other:

- Relatively high failure rate among perfect and typical users and does not protect against transmission of HIV, GC or chlamydia (see p. 152 - statement from 2002 CDC STI Treatment Guidelines). Spermicides may, in women having frequent intercourse with multiple partners, enhance transmission of HIV by irritation of vaginal mucosa and by destroying vaginal flora, e.g., lactobacilli, in nonoxynol-9 concentrations as low as 0.1% *[Van Dame, Durban, 2000 found 1.7 RR of HIV transmission in users of spermicidal vaginal gel with 52.5 mg N-9] [Kreiss - 1992]*
- Allergic reactions and dermatitis in women and men that could decrease compliance

COMPLICATIONS
- Women and men have confused fruit jelly, e.g., grape jelly, for spermicidal "jelly"
- Women and men have attempted to use cosmetics or hair products containing non-spermicidal octoxynols and nonoxynols (nonoxynol 4, 10, 12, and 14) in lieu of nonoxynol-9

CANDIDATES FOR USE
- Willing to accept high failure rates
- Any woman and partner who presents with no prior allergy or reaction to spermicides

Adolescents:
- Readily available and not contraindicated for teens unless at high risk for HIV infection
- High failure rate may discourage long-term use as primary method

INITIATING METHOD
- Except in cases where the patient, or partner, presents with pregnancy, allergy, or irritation, women can begin these methods at any time following product instructions
- Provide ECPs in advance

INSTRUCTIONS FOR PATIENT
- Inserting person should wash and dry hands
- Spermicide has its greatest efficacy near the cervical os
- Water exposure, e.g. bathing or douching, within 6 hours after insertion or post-coitally can minimize effectiveness; reapply before next penetrative act
- Keep spermicides in cool, dry places; tablets or foam can tolerate heat, film melts at 98.6° F

Creams/foams/gels
- Apply less than 1 hour prior to sexual intercourse. May drip out of vagina if inserted more than 1 hour in advance. With foam, shake canister vigorously. Fill plastic applicator with spermicide. Insert applicator deeply into vagina and depress plunger. Immediately active. Finish sexual intercourse within 60 minutes of application

Film, suppositories and tablets
- Insert at least 15 minutes before sexual intercourse: with film, fold the sheet in quarters and then half again (this aids insertion). Using fingers or an applicator, the inserting partner places the spermicide applicator or film deep in the vagina, near cervix. Finish sexual intercourse within 60 minutes of application

FOLLOW-UP
- Have you or your partner(s) experienced any rash or discomfort after using spermicides?
- Have you changed partners since beginning spermicides?
- Have you had sex—even once—without using spermicides?
- Would you like a more effective method?
- Did you have questions about ECPs? ◄
- Do you have Plan B emergency contraceptive pills in your medicine chest? ◄
- Do you plan to have children? OR Do you plan to have more children? If yes, when?

PROBLEM MANAGEMENT
Dermatitis: Discontinue spermicides and offer another method. If spermicide was used as lubricant, recommend a water-based or silicone-based lubricant without nonoxynol-9
Changed partners: Explain STI prevention, check for STIs, and recommend condoms

FERTILITY AFTER DISCONTINUATION OF METHOD
- No effect on baseline fertility

WILL THE SPONGE EVER RETURN?

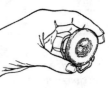

For thousands of years, women have placed sponges with a variety of spermicides into the vagina. The Today Contraceptive Sponge was going to be back on US pharmacy shelves by the end of 2001. Perhaps this will happen in 2006 or 2007. Call (201) 934-4449 for further information.

A recent Cochrane Review conducted by FHI found pregnancy rates during one year ◄ of sponge use to be 17% to 24% compared to 11% to 13% for the diaphragm *[Kuyoh MA-2003]*

To buy this book for students or staff, call **(706) 265-7435** or go to
www.managingcontraception.com

CHAPTER 23

Coitus Interruptus (Withdrawal)

www.managingcontraception.com

DESCRIPTION: Man withdraws penis completely from the vagina before ejaculation

EFFECTIVENESS

Perfect use failure rate in first year: 4% (See Trussell's failure rates, Table 13.2, p. 39)
Typical use failure rate in first year: 27%
[Trussell J IN Contraceptive Technology 2004]

MECHANISM: Withdrawal prior to ejaculation reduces or eliminates sperm introduced into vagina. Preejaculatory fluid is not generally a problem unless two acts of sexual intercourse are close together

Are there sperm in pre-ejaculate fluid? ←

Some concern exists that the pre-ejaculate fluid may carry sperm into the vagina. In itself, the pre-ejaculate, a lubricating secretion produced by the Littre or Cowper's glands, contains no sperm. Two studies examining the pre-ejaculate for the presence of spermatozoa found none. However, a previous ejaculation may have left some sperm hidden in the folds of the urethral lining. In examinations of the pre-ejaculate in one small study, the pre-ejaculate was free of spermatozoa in all of 11 HIV-seronegative men and 4 of 12 seropositive men. Although the 8 samples containing spermatozoa revealed only small clumps of a few hundred sperm, these could theoretically pose a risk of fertilization. In all likelihood, the spermatozoa left from a previous ejaculation could be washed out with the force of a normal urination; however, this remains unstudied. *[Kowal D. Coitus interruptus (withdrawal) IN Hatcher, RA Contraceptive Technology 18th edition. Page 314] [3 references]*

COST: None

ADVANTAGES

Menstrual: None
Sexual/psychological:
- No barriers
- Readily available method which encourages male involvement

Cancers, tumors, and masses: None
Other: Surprisingly effective if used correctly

DISADVANTAGES

Menstrual: None
Sexual/psychological
- May not be applicable for couples with sexual dysfunction such as premature ejaculation or unpredictable ejaculation
- Requires man's cooperation and instruction
- May reduce sexual pleasure of woman and intensity of orgasm of man
- Encourages "spectatoring" or thinking about what is happening during sexual intercourse

Cancers, tumors, and masses: None
Other: Relatively high failure rate among typical users and does not adequately protect against STIs. It may reduce risk of fluid-born infection

COMPLICATIONS: None

MEDICAL ELIGIBILITY CHECKLIST
- Man must be able to predict ejaculation in time to withdraw penis completely from vagina and move away from woman's external genetalia
- Premature ejaculation makes method less effective
- Appropriate for couples not at risk for STIs

CANDIDATES FOR USE
- Couples who are able to communicate during sexual intercourse
- Disciplined men who can ignore the powerful instinct, urging them to continue thrusting
- Couples in stable, mutually monogamous relationship
- Couples without religious or cultural prohibitions against withdrawal
- Women willing to accept higher risk of unintended pregnancy

Adolescents: Compliance may be a problem (as it is for couples of all ages); teens may have less control over ejaculation; advise use of condoms for better protection against pregnancy and STIs. While withdrawal is a relatively poor contraceptive option, especially if pregnancy prevention and infection control are very important, withdrawal is definitely better than using no contraceptive at all

INITIATING METHOD: Can begin at any time; provide ECPs in advance

INSTRUCTIONS FOR PATIENT
- Practice withdrawal using backup method until both partners master withdrawal
- Wipe penis clean of the pre-ejaculation fluid prior to vaginal penetration
- Use coital positions that ensure that the man will be capable of withdrawing easily at the appropriate time
- Use emergency contraception if withdrawal fails

FOLLOW-UP
- Does your partner ever ejaculate/begin to ejaculate before withdrawing?
- Do you want to use a more effective method?
- Did you have any Plan B in your medicine chest? ←
- Do you plan to have children? OR Do you plan to have more children?

PROBLEM MANAGEMENT
Failure to withdraw: Use ECPs everytime withdrawal does not work! Consider another method

FERTILITY AFTER DISCONTINUATION OF METHOD: No adverse effects on fertility (except the method does not adequately protect against STIs)

OVERVIEW: *Plan B should routinely be used as EC rather than combined pills*
The states with EC available direct from pharmacies are Washington, California, Alaska,
New Mexico, Hawaii and Maine. In 34 countries, EC is available directly from pharmacies.
Emergency contraception (EC) includes any method used after intercourse to prevent
pregnancy. None of the current methods is an abortifacient and none disturbs an implanted
pregnancy. There are currently 3 methods in widespread use worldwide:
• High-dose progestin-only contraceptive pills (POPs). PLAN B preferable to Ovrette or COCs
• (Yuzpe Method) 13 brands of combined oral contraceptive pills (COCs)
• Copper IUD insertion (Paragard)
An estimated 51,000 pregnancies were averted by EC use in 2000 accounting for 43% of the
decrease in abortions since 1994 *[Finer-2003]*. Only the two hormonal methods are utilized to
any significant degree in the U.S. (all combined and progestin-only pills that may be used are
on p. 86 of this book and in colored diagram on A-30). Provide ECPs to patients in advance in
one of 2 ways: give them pills in advance or give them a prescription with refills in advance

Table 24.1 Overview of Postcoital Methods Currently Available in U.S.

Characteristic	POPs	COCs *	Copper IUD
Timing of initiation after intercourse	ASAP but *can* be used up to 120 hours (5 days); Sooner is better	ASAP but *can* be used up to days 4 & 5 after unprotected sex; Sooner is better	Up to 8 days
Pregnancies/ 100 women	Early start: 0.4% (<12 h) Late start: 2.7% (1-3 days) Average: 1.1%	Early start: 0.5% (<12 h) Late start: 4.2% (1-3 days) Average: 2 - 3.2%	0.1%
Advantages	Fewer side effects than COCs; Product available for advance prescription: Plan B® **Both pills can be taken at once**	Wide range of COCs available for use	May be inserted 5 or more days after intercourse, but before implantation. Effective long-term contraceptive for appropriate women
Disadvantages	Less available than COCs that can be used to create an off-label EC regimen. Check for availability of Plan B at pharmacies near you at www.go2planb.com	Gastrointestinal side effects – can be reduced with antiemetic pretreatment No dedicated product	Expensive; must be appropriate candidate for IUD; Timing issues: counseling, testing, etc. Insertion procedure required
Side effects	Spotting. Same hormonal side effects as COCs, but less frequent and less severe	Nausea, vomiting, spotting headache, breast tenderness, moodiness, change in next menses	Pain, bleeding, expulsion
Avoid use in pregnant women and women with other prescribing precautions	Do not use in women with known pregnancy because the treatment will not be effective. Not a teratogen	Do not use in women with known pregnancy or current severe migraine. POPs are a better option for all women with a history of DVT or PE	Prescribing precautions for IUD use (see page 80)

For more information about EC, phone numbers of EC providers, or **to become listed as an EC provider**,
check out the web site www.not-2-late.com or call the EC Hotline at 1-888-NOT-2-LATE. Other good
sources of information about EC are www.go2planB.com or call 800-330-1271.

* COCs using norgestrel are better studied. COCs with norethindrone may be used as ECPs, but
failure rates are slightly higher as compared with COCs with norgestrel

How is NOR-Levo (France) different from Plan B (United States)?

NOR-Levo is the same postcoital pill as Plan B. Each is a progestin-only emergency contraceptive. Introduction of NOR-Levo in France in 1999 led quickly to a change in laws so that in 2002 NOR-Levo could be distributed free in middle and high schools. Minors can also obtain NOR-Levo free of charge in pharmacies without parental consent. Adult women can be reimbursed up to 65% of the cost of NOR-Levo by insurance. No adverse effects of NOR-Levo have been reported. The interest created by emergency contraception has created "more open discussion among pharmacists, nurses in schools and across all society about what to do to prevent pregnancy and sexually transmitted disease." (AGI 2003) France has one of the lowest abortion rates in the world: 12 per 1000 women aged 14-44 (AGI).

Contrast the above picture with the Plan B story in the United States. Approved at the end of the 1990s Plan B distribution is spotty at best. Many pharmacies do not stock Plan B. It requires a prescription in every state except Washington, California, Hawaii and New Mexico. No high schools or middle schools give it to students. And Plan B may cost anywhere from $10 to over $100. The current requirement to obtain Plan B increase the time from unprotected sex until Plan B is taken or lead to its not being used at all. In contrast to France, where discussion of emergency contraception has fostered increased discussion (and presumably use) of other contraceptives, controversy over emergency contraceptive pills has fueled debate in Kentucky and Ohio over how pills, mini-pills and Depo-Provera injections work jeopardizing the availability of these traditional contraceptives in the public family planning clinics of Northern Kentucky.

And the result: abortion rates in U.S. teens aged 15-19 are 3 times higher (29.2 vs. 10.2/1000) in the U.S. than in France and pregnancies in U.S. teens are 4 times higher (83.6 vs. 20.2) per 1000 teens in the U.S. than in France.

What is wrong with this picture? What seems to underscore the differences in how the United States and France approach teen sexuality - specifically how they approach sexual intercourse in teenagers.

Parents, teachers and community leaders in France and throughout Europe seem to be able to express the sentiment: "a teenager who is having intercourse must be responsible about this potentially dangerous activity."

Why is it that we can say to a 20 year-old who is drinking illegally "if you drink, don't drive?" Or a parent can say to his or her child, "if you drink, call me and I'll come get you." Parents, schools and public health facilities do not condone or encourage under-age drinking but do tell teens what to do if they drink. Similarly, parents, schools and public health facilties do not condone or encourage young teenagers to have intercourse and should be willing to tell teens what to do if they have unprotected intercourse exposing them to risk of pregnancy or sexually transmitted infections.

So, NOR-Levo and Plan B are exactly the same drug but France and the United States are as different as night and day in the access women have to this drug.

 Try calling 1-888-NOT 2 LATE and find out what women in you area-code learn about the 5 clinicians nearest to them who will help them with EC. You can sign up, too.

EMERGENCY CONTRACEPTION WITH EMERGENCY CONTRACEPTIVE PILLS

DESCRIPTION

POPs: more effective than COCs and less side effects

- Research indicates both tablets can be taken together in a single dose without significant reduction in efficacy or increase in side effects
- Both Plan B tabs or 1.5 mg of norgestrel at once OR in divided doses, take first dose ASAP within 120 hours after inadequately protected sex; take second dose 12 hours later (second dose may be more than 120 hours after unprotected sex). Second dose may also be taken less than 12 hours after the first dose
- Plan B is the only currently-available FDA-approved progestin-only product with instructions and pills that facilitate advance prescription
- Ovrette (20 yellow pills for each dose; she needs 2 packs of Ovrette)

Yuzpe Method using any of the levonorgestrel-containing COCs:

- Two large doses of COCs with at least 100 μg of ethinyl estradiol and either 100 mg of norgestrel or 50 mg of levonorgestrel in each dose. Norethindrone pills have slightly less effectiveness as ECPs. Take first dose ASAP within 72 hours after inadequately protected sex; take second dose 12 hours later (second dose may be taken up to 120 hours after unprotected sex). Try to provide ECPs to women in advance (actual pills or prescription with refills) (see Figure 24.1, p. 86)
- This approach is less effective and has more side effects than Plan B

EFFECTIVENESS

A randomized WHO trial of two levonorgestrel regimens (using LNG pills that were the same as Plan B tablets) found that taking 2 Plan B tablets at once was as effective (failure rate 1.5%) as taking 1 Plan B tablet followed by a second in 12 hours (failure rate 1.8%). The levonorgestrel dose need NOT be split. Both Plan B tablets may be taken at once without an increase in nausea (15%) or vomiting (1%). In this large trial, starting treatment with a delay of 4-5 days did not significantly increase the failure rate compared to the efficacy of treatment begun within 3 days of unprotected intercourse. *[von Hertzen-2002].* Failure rate was slightly higher when ECPs were taken on days 4 or 5. **Emergency contraceptive pills should be taken as soon as possible after unprotected sex**

EC with POPs PLAN B	Only 1.1% of 967 women using POPs for EC became pregnant in a WHO multi-center study *[WHO task force on Postovulatory Methods of Fertility Regulation. Lancet Aug 8, 1998].*	89% average reduction of pregnancy rate based on WHO perfect-use study population	12 pregnancies per 1000 unprotected acts of sexual intercourse followed by Plan B
EC with COCs	2-3% failure rate	74% average reduction of pregnancy rate (WHO perfect-use study)	20-32 pregnancies per 1000 unprotected acts of sexual intercourse followed by Preven or COCs

- Taking more than number of pills specified is *not* beneficial and may increase risk of vomiting

Plan B and other emergency contraceptive pills are NOT recommended for routine use as a contraceptive

MECHANISMS

- ECPs act by preventing pregnancy and never by disrupting an implanted pregnancy, i.e. never as an abortifacient
- If taken before ovulation, ECPs disrupt normal follicular development and maturation, blocks LH surge, and inhibit ovulation; they may also create deficient luteal phase and may have a contraceptive effect by thickening cervical mucus
- If taken after ovulation, ECPs have little effect on ovarian hormonal production and limited effect on endometrial maturation
- ECPs may affect tubal transport of sperm or ova

COST

POPs:
- Plan B is available in selected retail pharmacies for about $25 to $35.
- Ovrette (2 packs) is not readily available in all pharmacies and can cost up to $70
- Non-profit and Title X agencies may purchase Plan B at $4.50 - $8.00 per treatment
- Pharmacists in those states that may dispense without a prescription charge $50-$55 for counseling and medication

Yuzpe method with COCs:
- One cycle of COCs may vary from a few dollars to more than $50

Other costs:
- Cost prior to obtaining pills may vary from nothing (if already given) to cost of full exam and pregnancy test. This may increase total cost of EC to $45 to over $100

ADVANTAGES

Menstrual: None
Sexual/Psychological:
- Offers an opportunity to prevent pregnancy after rape, mistake, or overt barrier method failure (condom breaks or slips, diaphragm dislodges, etc.)
- Reduces anxiety about unintended pregnancy prior to next menses
- Process of getting EC may lead woman to initiate ongoing contraception

Cancers, tumors and masses: None
Other:
- There are 3 million unintended pregnancies each year; nearly half of all pregnancies are unintended. *[Henshaw, 1998]* Widespread availability of ECPs could halve the number of unintended pregnancies and the consequent need for abortion [Trussell, 1992]
- 40% of reduction in teen pregnancies ('95 to '99) due to EC
- Could reduce birth defects (poor use of folic acid if conception is not planned)
- Reduces ectopic pregnancy rate

DISADVANTAGES

Menstrual:
- Next menses may be early (especially if taken before ovulation), on time, or late
- Notable changes in flow of next menses seen in 10-15% of women
- **If no menses within 3 weeks (21 days) of taking ECPs, pregnancy test should be done**

Sexual/psychological:
- Women who are uncomfortable with post-fertilization methods might need reassurance that use of EC with COCs or POPs is consistent with their beliefs if taken during the follicular phase. They also may need to be warned that if taken after ovulation, ECPs may work as an interceptive (ie prevent implantation of fertilized egg)

Cancers, tumors and masses: None

Other:

- Breast tenderness, fatigue, headache, abdominal pain and dizziness
- No protection against STIs; consider treatment for possible STIs following exposure
- Many pharmacies do not carry Plan B. Physicians and nurse practitioners wanting to overcome this problem can do 2 things:
  1. Write prescriptions and encourage women to buy Plan B in advance ◄
  2. Hand notes to their paitents requesting that pharmacists keep Plan B in stock ◄

Nausea and vomiting:

	Nausea	Vomiting	Pretreatment with antiemetic
POPs (Plan B)	23%	6%	Many clinicians use only if Hx of past problems with nausea or vomiting
COCs	50%	19%	Can reduce symptoms by 30-50%

COMPLICATIONS

- Several cases of DVT reported in women using COCs as ECPs. No increased DVT risk with POPs

CANDIDATES FOR USE

Some clinicians provide Plan B to men so they will have it ready if their partner needs it ◄

- All women who have had or who may be at risk for unprotected sex (sperm exposure) are candidates for ECPs for immediate or future use. Women with strong contraindications to estrogen use should use POPs (see **PRESCRIBING PRECAUTIONS**)
- As a backup method for barrier methods
- There are many situations in which women have unintended sperm exposure:
  - Failed contraceptive methods: broken condom, dislodged diaphragm, or cervical cap, forgotten pills, late for contraceptive reinjection, NFP miscalculation, failed withdrawal
  - Failure to use methods: clouded judgment, passion, sexual assault
- For the woman who has intercourse infrequently (1-2x/yr) Particularly effective if taken within one hour of otherwise unprotected sex
- NOTE: ECPs do not protect against pregnancy as well as ongoing methods

Adolescents: appropriate back-up option (**definitely provide ECPs in advance to all teens**). Having EC available does NOT make teens less likely to use regular contraception or more likely to have unprotected sex. *[Glasier-1998] [Raine-2000] [Ellertson-2001]* ◄

PRECAUTIONS

Plan B:

- Pregnancy (no benefit; no effect)
- Hypersensitivity to any component of product
- Undiagnosed abnormal vaginal bleeding
- No STI protection

Use of COCs for EC should be allowed for all women except those who:

- Are pregnant; no benefit but also no dangers
- Are known to be hypersensitive to any component of the product
- Have acute migraine headaches at the time ECPs are to be taken (Use Plan B)
- Have history of DVT or PE (use POPs - Plan B)

INITIATING METHOD: Pregnancy testing is optional, not required:

- Offer ECPs routinely to all women who may be at risk for unprotected intercourse: Plan B (levonorgestrel) is better than combined pills
  - Advance prescription increases use of EC but does not diminish use of primary method of contraception
  - Availability directly through pharmacists led to a thousand-fold increase in use of ECPs in selected pharmacies in the state of Washington
- Provide EC for all women who present after-the-fact, acutely in need. If you dispense off-label pills remove the inactive pills to reduce risk of mistake
- Patient history for prescribing EC after-the-fact:
  - LMP, previous menstrual period, dates of any prior unprotected intercourse this cycle, and date and time of last unprotected intercourse
  - Any problems with previous use of ECPs, COCs or POPs?
  - Breast-feeding or severe headaches now? History of DVT or PE? (Use Plan B not COCs)
  - Any foreseeable problems if antiemetic causes drowsiness?
- No physical exam/labs needed on a routine basis:
  - No pelvic exam is necessary, now or in the past; No BP measurements needed
  - Pregnancy testing useful only if concerned that prior intercourse may have caused pregnancy. *ACOG, IPPF and WHO do not include routine pregnancy testing in their protocols*
- Advise patient about possible side effects and consider other EC options (Copper IUD)
- If prescribing COCs, offer premedication with long-acting antiemetic one hour prior to first ECP dose. Take two 25 mg tablets of meclizine hydrochloride (over-the-counter Dramamine or Bonine). Other agents work, but do not have same duration of action. Avoid antiemetic if drowsiness will pose safety hazard. Antiemetics not needed prior to Plan B
- Tell her how to use appropriate number of tablets for particular ECP brand to reach adequate dose (see Figure 24.1, p. 86 and p. A-30 opposite inside back cover).
- **Both Plan B tabs may be taken at once.** If using COCs, encourage patient to take first dose ASAP and second dose approximately 12 hours after first dose. It is ok to take second dose in slightly less or more than 12 hours; realize that 72 hours is NOT the absolute limit. ECP may be taken for up to 120 hours after unprotected sex
- Consider providing EC now for patient to have available at home in case she has another need to use EC again OR provide prescription with refills
- Inquire about desire to be checked for STI's (especially in cases of rape)

STARTING REGULAR USE OF CONTRACEPTIVE AFTER USE OF ECPs

- Start using regular method immediately. ECPs offer no lingering reliable protection
- If missed OCs, restart day after ECPs taken (no need to catch up missed pills)
- If starting COCs, patch or ring, see COC precautions and then:
  - May wait for next menses or
  - Start OCs, patch or ring next day with 7-day backup method (this will affect timing of next menses). In office she may punch out a few pills at the beginning of a pill pack to correspond with the date you are seeing her. This may reduce confusion
- If starting DMPA injections, can start immediately. If so, consider having patient return in 2-3 weeks for pregnancy test
- If starting barrier methods, start immediately.
- If starting NFP, use abstinence (or barrier/spermicide) until next menses

SPECIAL ISSUES/FREQUENT QUESTIONS

- Give your patient a supply (3 Plan B packs) of EC at her annual visit. EC is more likely ◄
  to be used if she already has it and need not visit a pharmacy *(Glasier 2001; Jackson 2003; Raine 2005)*
- When in cycle should EC be offered? Anytime except perhaps if she is having her menses
- How many times a year can a woman use ECPs? No limit, but be sure to ask her why
  her primary method is not working
- What if a patient has had unprotected intercourse earlier in the cycle? Do urine test to
  confirm no obvious pregnancy. Offer EC. If concerned that your test may miss an early
  pregnancy, give EC and have her return in 3 weeks (if no menses) for another pregnancy
  test. EC will not adversely affect the fetus or a pregnancy
- What if she used EC earlier in the month? Offer it again; she may have just delayed
  ovulation. Review why her primary contraceptive is failing and remedy the situation
  (perhaps with a new method). Consider performing pregnancy test in this setting even
  though it may be too early to have become positive; counsel her about this possibility
- What if the pharmacy is closed or does not carry EC? Plan ahead—provide EC by advance
  prescription. Check with local 24-hour pharmacies; encourage stocking up with Plan B.
  Also visit www.go2planb.com
- What if a woman whom I have not seen previously calls for ECPs? Some practitioners
  screen over the telephone and telephone in prescriptions to pharmacies. In some states,
  the law requires face to face contact to establish physician-patient relationship

INSTRUCTIONS FOR PATIENT

- **EC works best if taken as soon as possible after sex. Each woman needs Plan B in** ◄
  her medicine chest! For advance prescription, have her fill her prescription (or obtain
  OTC in advance) and keep readily available. Approved shelf life of Plan B is said in U.S.
  packaging to be 18 months! However, the approved shelf life in Europe for exactly the same
  medication is stated to be 5 years.
- **It is now recommended that both doses of Plan B be taken at once** ◄
- An antiemetic need *not* be taken prior to Plan B
- Start using contraception right away. ECPs do not reliably protect you beyond the day
  they are used
- Re-evaluate primary contraceptive method to make it more reliable
- Have her return for pregnancy testing if she has not had her menses 21 days after using ECPs

FOLLOW-UP

- No routine follow-up needed
- Have patient return for pregnancy testing if no menses in 3 weeks

PROBLEM MANAGEMENT

Nausea/vomiting:

- Plan B is preferable to combined hormonal pills as EC, because Plan B is more effective ◄
  and has a lower risk of both nausea and vomiting (see p. 81)
- Antiemetic may be prescribed before or after taking combined COCs as ECPs (does not
  work as well when taken after EC)
- Vomiting that occurs due to ECPs probably indicates that enough hormones reached the
  bloodstream to have the desired contraceptive effect. Most experts (but NOT all) recommend
  a repeat dose of ECPs if vomiting occurs within 30 minutes of taking ECPs. ACOG
  recommends a repeat dose if vomiting occurs within one hour *[ACOG 1996]*

- Plan B is preferable to COCs, but if repeating dose because of severe vomiting, switch from COCs to POPs or consider placing pills in vagina rather than mouth (off-label). Although uptake is slower, this may also be possible for woman who has experienced extreme nausea while taking COCs in the past as her regular contraceptive. No data on effectiveness of vaginal COCs used as EC
- If severe vomiting occurs, consider IUD as emergency contraceptive

Amenorrhea:
- If menses do not occur in 21 days (or more than 7 days beyond expected day for menses to begin), need to rule out pregnancy. Pregnancy test recommended

Pregnancy in spite of using ECPs:
- If there is a pregnancy, the woman may be reassured that there is evidence that ECPs do not increase the risk of fetal anomalies or miscarriage

FERTILITY AFTER DISCONTINUATION OF METHOD

Must provide contraception for rest of cycle and beyond. If she starts using birth control pills or a vaginal ring, use a back-up (condoms) for the first 7 days. If she uses patches, use a back-up (condoms) for 9 days

EMERGENCY CONTRACEPTION WITH COPPER IUD

DESCRIPTION

- Insert Copper IUD, following the usual procedures, within 5 days after unprotected or inadequately protected sexual intercourse. May be used up to 8 days after intercourse, if ovulation is known to have occurred 3 days or more after the unprotected sex
- More frequently used overseas, where IUD costs are lower
- In the US, this method is generally restricted to use by women who intend to continue to use the IUD as an ongoing method
- Levonorgestrel IUD (Mirena) is definitely NOT indicated for use as EC

EFFECTIVENESS

- **Definitely the most effective postcoital contraceptive**
- Failure rate < 1% (only about 6 pregnancies per 1000 insertions in world's literature)

MECHANISM

- In the month it is inserted as an emergency contraceptive, it may act by interfering with implantation (see pages 88 and 96 for mecchanisms of action of IUDs as routine, long-term contraceptive

COST

- In U.S. about $500. In Europe postcoital IUD insertion costs just $25 (Belgium) or is covered by health plan. Inexpensive in Europe or in the United States in comparison with costs (emotional and financial) of an unintended pregnancy

ADVANTAGES

- The most effective post-coital method and may be used 2-5 days later than ECPs
- Provides long-term protection against pregnancy following insertion

DISADVANTAGES: Same as using Copper IUD as contraceptive (See Chapter 25, p. 88-100)
- Very expensive, if only used for EC and removal expected soon
- Timing constraints of EC use may make it difficult to properly screen patients for IUD insertion (counseling, preinsertion cultures, etc.)

COMPLICATIONS, CANDIDATES FOR USE, PRESCRIBING PRECAUTIONS, INITIATING METHOD, INSTRUCTIONS FOR PATIENT FOLLOW-UP, PROBLEM MANAGEMENT, FERTILITY AFTER USE
- Same as using Copper IUD as ongoing contraceptive (See Chapter 25, p. 88-100)

EMERGENCY CONTRACEPTION WITH MIFEPRISTONE (RU-486)

DESCRIPTION
- Single 10 mg to 25 mg dose of the anti-progestogen mifepristone (RU-486), taken within 5 days of unprotected intercourse. Not available in the United States. Still not approved by any major regulatory agency in the world

EFFECTIVENESS
- About the same effectiveness as levonorgestrel (Plan B) in most recent study *[Lancet-12/7/02]*
- One international study allowed initiation up to 120 hours and still found 85% overall efficacy

MECHANISMS
- Blocks action of progesterone by binding to its receptors
- Stops ovulation if given in follicular phase (contraceptive)
- Slows endometrial maturation in luteal phase (interceptive)

FERTILITY AFTER DISCONTINUATION OF METHOD
- Fertility may return later in cycle or with next menses

 Try calling 1-888-NOT 2 LATE and find out what women in you area-code learn about the 5 clinicians nearest to them who will help them with EC. You can sign up, too.

To order *Managing Contraception* or the 18th edition of *Contraceptive Technology*, call (706) 265-7435 or go to **www.managingcontraception.com**

Figure 24.1

EMERGENCY CONTRACEPTION USING EMERGENCY CONTRACEPTIVE PILLS (ECPs)

1-888-NOT-2 LATE; www.opr.princeton.edu/ec; www.go2planB.com

Prescribe/provide emergency contraceptive pills (ECPs) **prior to the need** for them so that women and men have them available at home (or rapid access to them) in case they are needed. This is particularly important since some pharmacies will not dispense ECPs

---

Start ECPs as soon as possible, after unprotected or inadequately protected sexual intercourse. **Can be used up to 5 days, but sooner is better; most effective if taken immediately or within 12 hours**

No need to use anti-nausea medication if using Plan B. If using a COC, first, take anti-nausea medication: 50 mg oral meclizine* has 24-hour duration of action

---

BRAND**	DOSE
Plan B	2 white tablets all at once***
Ovrette	20 yellow tablets

One hour after antiemetic, take first dose of ECPs. Choose one of the following:

Ogestrel, Ovral	2 white tablets	
Levora, Low-Ogestrel, Lo/Ovral	4 white tablets	If vomiting occurs within 1 hour, repeat dose
Levlen, Nordette	4 light-orange tablets	
Tri-Levlen, Triphasil	4 light-yellow tablets	
Trivora	4 pink tablets	
Alesse, Levlite	5 pink tablets	

CALL: 1-888-NOT-2 LATE if you have any questions about emergency contraception OR if you need to hear about EC in Spanish or if you need phone numbers of 5 clinicians nearest you who will provide EC.

If using one of the other COC options, repeat the same dose of ECPs 12 hours later. In the case of Plan B, both tabs may be taken at once

---

Patient should (re)start ongoing method immediately and restock Plan B at home

---

Pregnancy test if no period in 3 weeks

NOTE: if anti-nausea medication is NOT taken prior to first dose of ECPs (which is recommended), it may be taken after the first dose, should nausea be severe or should woman vomit. Anti-nausea medication is usually not needed for women using PLAN B, as PLAN B does not contain estrogen

* Meclizine hydrochloride is recommended because it has a 24-hour duration of action. It is available over the counter as Bonine and as Dramamine 2. Other medications to prevent nausea may be prescribed instead.

**Norethindrone pills recently shown to be effective

***Labeling recommends one tablet now and one in 12 hours, but new studies show that taking 2 tablets at once is equally effective (and more convenient). Two Plan B tablets ASAP within ← 5 days is becoming the instruction for women using Plan B

Figure 24.2

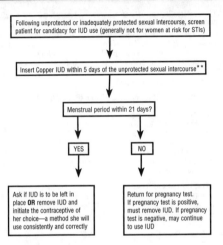

EMERGENCY CONTRACEPTION USING COPPER IUD*
www.opr.princeton.edu/ec

Following unprotected or inadequately protected sexual intercourse, screen patient for candidacy for IUD use (generally not for women at risk for STIs)

↓

Insert Copper IUD within 5 days of the unprotected sexual intercourse**

↓

Menstrual period within 21 days?

YES → Ask if IUD is to be left in place **OR** remove IUD and initiate the contraceptive of her choice—a method she will use consistently and correctly

NO → Return for pregnancy test. If pregnancy test is positive, must remove IUD. If pregnancy test is negative, may continue to use IUD

* There is no evidence that Mirena, the levonorgestrel IUS, is effective for EC

** The Copper IUD may be inserted up to the time of implantation—about 5 days after ovulation—to prevent pregnancy. Thus, if a woman had unprotected sexual intercourse 3 days before ovulation occurred in that cycle, the IUD could be inserted up to 8 days after intercourse to prevent pregnancy

Postcoital ParaGard insertion is the most effective emergency contraceptive. If a woman can use a Copper T 380 A IUD as her emergency contraceptive and leave it in as her ongoing long-term contraceptive, she may receive 10 or more years of excellent contraceptive protection.

 CALL: 1-888-NOT-2 LATE if you have any questions about emergency contraception OR if you need to hear about EC in Spanish or if you need phone numbers of 5 clinicians nearest you who will provide EC.

CHAPTER 25

Intrauterine Contraceptives
www.popcouncil.org, www.engenderhealth.org,
www.berlex.com, www.arhp.org

OVERVIEW: A Johns Hopkins webpage has pictures of many IUDs. Go to **www.jhuccp. org/pr/b6/b6used.stm** The only two intrauterine contraceptives available in the U.S. are the ParaGard® T 380A Intrauterine Copper IUD and the Mirena® levonorgestrel-releasing intrauterine system (LNG-IUS). For intrauterine contraception to play the role it could play, clinicians must become more supportive of the role of insertion immediately following abortion AND younger women and never-pregnant women should NOT be excluded from using IUDs. Post-placental IUD insertion is another practice that could lead to more use of IUDs/IUCs in the United States (see page 92)

INTRAUTERINE COPPER CONTRACEPTIVE (ParaGard T 380A)

DESCRIPTION: T-shaped intrauterine contraceptive made of
radiopaque polyethylene, with two flexible arms that bend down for insertion
but open in the uterus to hold solid sleeves of copper against fundus.
Fine copper wire wrapped around stem. Surface area of copper = 380 mm^2.
Monofilament polyethylene tail string threaded through and knotted below
blunt ball at base of stem creates double strings that protrude into vagina.
This IUD has 2 straw colored strings

EFFECTIVENESS: *Think of IUDs/IUCs as "reversible sterilization"*
• Approved for 10 years use; effective for 12 years at least
Perfect use failure rate in first year: 0.6% (see Table 13.2, p. 38)
Typical use failure rate in first year: 0.8%
[Trussell J IN Contraceptive Technology, 2004]
Cumulative 10-year failure rate: 2.1 - 2.8%

MECHANISMS
The intrauterine copper contraceptive works primarily as a spermicide. Copper ions inhibit sperm motility and acrosomal enzyme activation so that sperm rarely reach the fallopian tube and are unable to fertilize the ovum. The sterile inflammatory reaction created in the endometrium phagocytizes the sperm. Experimental evidence suggests that the IUDs do not routinely work after fertilization. They are not abortifacients. They primarily prevent pregnancy by killing sperm (spermicidal), and then preventing fertilization

COST: From $0 to well over $500

ADVANTAGES: Effective long-term contraception from a single decision
Menstrual: none
Sexual/psychological
• Convenient; permits spontaneous sexual activities. Requires no action at time of use
• Intercourse may be more pleasurable with risk of pregnancy reduced
Cancers, tumors and masses
• Probable protection against endometrial cancer (6 of 7 case control studies)
  [Hubacher-Grimes-2002]
• Possible 40% protection against cervical cancer *[Grimes-2004]*

Other
- Rapid return to fertility and private
- Convenient - single insertion provides up to 12 years protection (package labeling says 10 years)
- **Cost effective. Provides greatest net benefits of any contraceptive over a 5 year period.**
- Good option for women who cannot use hormonal methods
- Risk for ectopic pregnancy decreased to 1/10th the risk
- **IUDs lead to highest level of user satisfaction, 99%, of any contraceptive currently being used by women** *[Forrest-1996]*

Menstrual
- Average monthly blood loss increased by about 35%; this may be diminished by NSAIDs
- May increase dysmenorrhea (removal rates for bleeding and pain first year = 11.9%)
- Spotting and cramping with insertion and intermittently in weeks following insertion

Sexual/psychological
- Some women uncomfortable with concept of having "something" (foreign body) placed inside them
- Some women are not at ease checking strings
- Strings palpable; if strings cut too short, may cause partner discomfort

Cancers, tumors and masses: None

Other
- Requires office procedure for insertion and removal; both can be uncomfortable
- Some programs/protocols recommend a chlamydia/gc check before insertion, others do not
- Some do a wet mount with cultures. If bacterial vaginosis or trichomonas, may still ◄ insert IUD and start treatment on the same visit (WHO 2004 MEC)
- Increases risk of infection in first 20 days after insertion (1/1000 women will get PID)
- Offers no protection from HIV/STIs; PID: see data in box below
- May be expelled obviously (with cramping and bleeding) or silently (unknowingly placing woman at risk for pregnancy). Rate of expulsion declines over time. At 5 years cumulative expulsion rate (partial or complete) is 11.3%. Expulsion rate for the 5th year is 0.3%. Women who have expelled one IUD have about a one in three chance of expelling an IUD if another is inserted *[Grimes-2004]*

COMPLICATIONS: See PROBLEM MANAGEMENT section for details

Complication	Frequency	Risk factors
PID within 20 days	1/1000	BV, cervicitis, contamination with insertion
Uterine perforation	1/1000	Immobile, markedly verted uterus Breast-feeding woman Inexperienced, unskilled inserter
Vasovagal reaction or Fainting with insertion	Rare	Stenotic os, pain Prior vasovagal reaction
Expulsion		Insertion on menses, immediately postpartum, not high enough in fundus or nulliparous
Pregnancy		Poor placement, expulsion

CANDIDATES FOR USE: *Think of IUDs as reversible sterilization*

• See 2004 WHO Medical Eligibility Criteria, pages A-1 through A-8
• Currently recommended patient profile includes women in stable mutually monogamous relationships (at low risk of STIs). The copper IUD and LNG IUD are best for women seeking longer-term (≥ 2 years) pregnancy protection due to their high initial cost
• Nulligravid women at low risk for STIs may also be candidates
• Women with history of PID may be candidates if they are currently have no known risk ◄ factors for STIs
• Good option for women who cannot or do not want to use hormones
Adolescents: Adolescents usually do not meet all the criteria for IUD use and may not tolerate increased bleeding and cramping with menses caused by the Copper IUD

PRESCRIBING PRECAUTIONS: See WHO Eligibility Criteria, **pages A1-A8**
• Pregnancy
• Uterus < 6 cm or > 9 cm (package insert, but may be able to use if >9 cm. Some clinicians use an upper limit of 10-12 cm)
• Undiagnosed abnormal vaginal bleeding
• Severe anemia (relative contraindication) (levonorgestrel IUD would be a good choice)
• Active cervicitis or active pelvic infection or known symptomatic actinomycosis
• Women with current STI, STI within 3 months or women at risk (multiple sex partners)
• Recent endometritis (last 3 months); See WHO recommendations, A-6
• Allergy to copper; Wilson's disease
• Uterine anomaly or fibroid(s) distorting uterine cavity (WHO 2004) preventing even ◄ distribution of copper ions or fundal placement of IUD
• AIDS (WHO: 3), HIV-infected (WHO: 2), AIDS, clinically well on antiretroviral therapy ◄ (WHO: 2), high risk of HIV (WHO: 2) IUD's do not increase complications in women with HIV/AIDS *[Curtis - 2002]*
• Known or suspected uterine or cervical CA - Insertion (WHO: 4), continuation (WHO: 2) ◄

INITIATING METHOD
• Requires insertion by trained professional
• May be inserted at any time in cycle when pregnancy can be ruled out; lowest overall rates of expulsion are when insertion is at midcycle
• May be inserted immediately after induced, therapeutic or first trimester spontaneous abortion if infection can be ruled out (increased risk of expulsion if > 9 weeks)
• May be inserted immediately after delivery of the placenta or prior to discharge from hospital after delivery or may await complete uterine involution postpartum or following second or third trimester loss (increased risk of expulsion)
• One IUD may be removed and a second inserted at the same visit
• Test for cervical infection, if indicated. Rule out BV; can start BV or trichomonas Rx ◄ and insert IUD the same day (WHO 2004)

INSERTION TIPS: Each step should be performed slowly and gently
• All clinicians wanting to insert IUDs would benefit from training in IUD insertion
• Reconfirm formal consent; Give NSAIDs one hour prior to insertion
• Be sure patient is not pregnant
• Routine antibiotic prophylaxis is not warranted; American Heart Association requires **no** antibiotic treatment except for women at high risk for bacterial endocarditis
• Recheck position, size and mobility of uterus prior to insertion
• Cleanse upper vaginal, outer cervix, and cervical os and canal thoroughly with antiseptic

- Local anesthesia at tenaculum site: 3 approaches are 1) no anesthesia 2) apply benzocaine 20% gel first at tenaculum site then leave a gel-soaked cotton-tipped applicator in cervical canal for 1 minute before proceeding with IUD insertion (Speroff/Darney p. 245) 3) inject 1 ml of local anesthetic (1% chloroprocaine) into the cervical lip into which the tenaculum will be placed
- Paracervical block at 3 and 9 o'clock: 2 approaches are 1) no anesthesia 2) 5 cc of local anesthetic on each side (more details Speroff/Darney text p. 245)
- Place tenaculum to stabilize cervix and straighten uterine axis.
- Sound uterus to fundus with uterine sound or pipelle; hold sound like a pencil when entering internal os to limit uterine perforation risk
- After insertion, trim strings to about 2" (5 cm). Mark length of strings on chart for later follow-up visits to confirm that length is the same
- If in doubt that IUD is at the fundus, e.g. after post-abortion or post-placental insertion, check with sonography

Figure 25.1 How to insert a Copper IUD

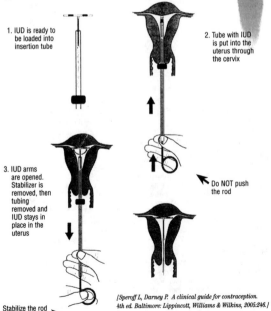

1. IUD is ready to be loaded into insertion tube

2. Tube with IUD is put into the uterus through the cervix

Do NOT push the rod

3. IUD arms are opened. Stabilizer is removed, then tubing removed and IUD stays in place in the uterus

Stabilize the rod with this hand

[Speroff L, Darney P. A clinical guide for contraception. 4th ed. Baltimore: Lippincott, Williams & Wilkins, 2005:246.]

POSTPLACENTAL & IMMEDIATE POSTPARTUM INSERTION

- Postplacental (preferably within 10 minutes after expulsion of the placenta) and immediate postpartum insertion during the first week after delivery (but preferably within 48 hours) are convenient effective and safe times to insert copper IUDs. Most studies have been performed in non-industrialized countries
- Expulsion rates of 7- 15% at 6 months require that women receiving an IUD very soon after delivery be told how to detect expulsions and instructed to return for reinsertion
- Unplanned pregnancy rates of post placental IUD insertion range from 2.0 - 2.8 per 100 users at 24 months *[O'Hanley-1992]*. After 1 year, one study found a failure rate of 0.8% following post-placental IUD insertion, comparable to interval insertions *[Thiery-1985]*
- The risk of infection is low following post-placental IUD insertion, with rates of 0.1% to 1.1% *[Lean-1967][Dharmeapanij-1970][Snidvongs-1970][Cole-1984]*. Rates of perforation are very low during post-placental IUD insertion, approximately 1 perforation in each study with patient populations ranging from 1150 to 3800 women *[Cole-1984][Edelman-1979][Phatak-1970]*

Figure 25.2 Two techniques of postplacental IUD insertion and proper location of IUD after insertion

A) IUD strings placed in palm of hand

B) Manual insertion at top of fundus

C) Use of ring forceps to insert IUD

INSTRUCTIONS FOR PATIENT

- Give patient trimmed IUD strings to learn what to check for after menses each month (strings may not be apparent until a few months after post-placental insertion)
- Advise patients to return if any symptoms of pregnancy, infection or IUD loss develop:

PAINS: *"Early IUD Warning Signs"*	
P	Period late (pregnancy); abnormal spotting or bleeding
A	Abdominal pain, pain with intercourse
I	Infection exposure (STI); abnormal vaginal discharge
N	Not feeling well, fever, chills
S	String missing, shorter or longer

- Counsel patient on anticipated menstrual changes. Ask *"Will a change in your menstrual bleeding pattern be acceptable to you?"* May take NSAIDs for first 2-3 days of next 3 menses (eg, ibuprofen 400 mg every 6 hours starting at beginning of flow).

FOLLOW-UP: Ask about risk for STIs. Provide condoms if at risk

- Have patient return for post-insertion check about 2 1/2 months after insertion to rule out partial expulsion or other problems requiring removal. Return earlier if any problems
- May be left in place during evaluation and treatment for cervical dysplasia
- Can you feel your IUD strings? Have they changed in length?
- Have you or your partner had any new partners since your last visit?

PROBLEM MANAGEMENT

Uterine perforation: All perforations occur or begin at insertion

- Clinical signs: pain, loss of resistance to advancement of instrument and instrument introduced deeper than uterus thought to be on bimanual exam
- Perforation by uterine sound usually occurs in midline posterior uterine wall when there is marked flexion:
  - Remove uterine sound
  - If no bleeding seen, stable BP and pulse, patient pain free and hematocrit stable for next several hours, she may be sent home. Provide alternate contraception
  - If any persistent pain or signs of other organ damage, take or refer immediately for laparoscopic evaluation (extremely rare)
- If IUD perforates acutely, attempt removal by gently pulling on strings
  - If resistance encountered, stop and do pelvic ultrasound and/or send to surgery for immediate laparoscopic IUD removal
- If IUD perforation noted and confirmed by ultrasound at later date, if asymptomatic, arrange for elective laparoscopic removal. Provide interval contraceptive. Can have IUD inserted later (i.e. not a contraindication to future IUDs) **◄**

Spotting, frequent or heavy bleeding, hemorrhage, anemia:

- Rule out pregnancy. If pregnant, rule out ectopic pregnancy
- Rule out infection, especially if post-coital bleeding
- Rule out expulsion or partial expulsion of IUD (see below)
- If anemic, provide iron supplement and deal with cause
- Offer NSAIDs every month to reduce bleeding
- Consider replacement with Mirena, the hormonal intrauterine contraceptive **◄**

Cramping and/or pain:

- Rule out pregnancy, infection, IUD expulsion
- Offer NSAIDs with menses or just before menses every month to reduce cramping
- Consider IUD removal and use of LNG IUD or another method if problem persists

Expulsion/partial expulsion:

- If expulsion confirmed (IUD seen by patient or clinician), rule out pregnancy. May place a new IUD
- If expulsion suspected, do ultrasound to determine IUD absence or presence and location. Probe endocervical canal for IUD, remove if not properly placed. May replace immediately if patient not pregnant
- If partial expulsion, remove IUD. If no infections and not pregnant, may replace with new IUD. If IUD not replaced, provide new contraceptive

Strings not felt:

- Check vagina for strings. Assess string length. If normal, reassure and re-instruct patient how to feel for strings
- If strings missing, do pregnancy test and ultrasound to determine if IUD has been expelled.

Missing strings in non-pregnant patients:

- Twist cytobrush inside cervix to snag strings which may have become snarled in canal
- Ultrasound to determine IUD presence and location **◄**
- If IUD in endocervix, remove and offer to replace
- If IUD not in cervical canal, IUD may be left in place or removed.
- If decision is made to remove IUD after paracervical block, attempt to remove with alligator forceps (some clinicians obtain informed consent after reviewing risks of procedure) or refer for ultrasound to localize prior to attempted removal (provide interim birth control). A 5mm Novak curette (much more painful than alligator forceps) and/or concurrent sonography may be useful in removal of IUDs. In non-pregnant patients, removal may also be done under ultrasound guidance or hysteroscopy

Missing strings in pregnant patients:
- Rule out ectopic pregnancy: 5-8% of all failures with the copper IUD are ectopic
- If intrauterine pregnancy, obtain ultrasound to verify IUD in situ
- If IUD is in uterus, advise patient she is at increased risk for preterm labor and spontaneous abortion but reassure her that fetus is not at increased risk for birth defects. May remove IUD at surgery if patient desires elective abortion. Otherwise, plan for removal at delivery

Pregnancy with visible strings:
- Visible strings in first trimester: advise removal of IUD to reduce risk of spontaneous abortion and premature labor
- Patient having miscarriage: Remove IUD. Consider antibiotics for 7 days

Infection with IUD use:
- *BV or candidiasis:* treat routinely
- *Trichomoniasis:* treat and reassess IUD candidacy
- *Cervicitis or PID:* Give first dose of antibiotics to achieve adequate serum levels before removing IUD. IUD removal not necessary unless no improvement after antibiotic Rx. Patient may not be candidate for continued IUD use. (WHO: 2 for continuation for both STI and PID)
- *Actinomycosis:* Culture of asymptomatic women without an IUD AND of women with an IUD both find that 3-4% are positive for Actinomyces *[Lippes, J. Am J Obstet Gyn-1999; 180-2 65-9]*. Often suggested by Pap smear report of "Actinomycosis-like organisms". True upper tract infection with this organism is very serious and requires at least prolonged IV antibiotic therapy with penicillin. However, less than half of women with such Pap smear reports have actinomyces and those that do usually have asymptomatic colonization only. Examine patient for any signs of PID (it can be unilateral). If signs of upper tract involvement Treat with antibiotics x 1 month. If patient has no clinical evidence of upper tract involvement, 3 options are available depending on patient's wishes and risk of infection: ◀
  1. Conservative. Annual pap smears only. Advise patient to return as needed or if she develops PID symptoms or
  2. Treat with antibiotic penicillin G (500 mg qid p.o. x 2 weeks) or a tetracycline(tetracycline 500 mg qid p.o. for a month OR doxycycline 100 mg bid x 2 weeks) and repeat Pap smear or
  3. Remove IUD, treat with antibiotic, and repeat Pap smear in 1 month. Reinsert if colonization cleared

REMOVAL

Indications: Expelling IUD, infection, pregnant, expired IUD, complications with IUD, anemia, no longer candidate for IUD, patient request.
Procedure: Grasp the strings close to external os and steadily retract until IUD removed
Complications
- Embedded IUD: Gentle rotation of strings may free IUD. If still stuck, may use alligator forceps removal with or without sonographic guidance (see Missing strings, p. 83). Hysteroscopic removal may be indicated in rare cases. A paracervical block reduces pain from removal of an embedded IUD
- Broken strings: Remove IUD with alligator forceps or Novak curette (much more painful)

FERTILITY AFTER DISCONTINUATION OF METHOD
Immediate return to baseline fertility

LEVONORGESTREL INTRAUTERINE SYSTEM (Mirena®)

DESCRIPTION: T-shaped intrauterine contraceptive placed within uterine cavity that initially releases 20 micrograms/day of levonorgestrel from its vertical reservoir. Release falls to 14 mcg per day after 5 years. Product information/ordering: 1-866-647-3646. IUD has 2 gray strings

EFFECTIVENESS: Effective for up to 5 years (label)
Perfect use failure rate in first year: 0.1% (See Table 13.2, p. 38)
Typical use failure rate in first year: 0.1% *[Trussell J. IN Contraceptive Technology, 2004]*
5-year cumulative failure rate: 0.7%
7-year cumulative failure rate: 1.1% *[Sivin-1991]*
• 1-year continuation rate in Finland: 93%; 2 years: 87% *[Bachman-BJOG, 2000]*

MECHANISM: Levonorgestrel causes cervical mucus to become thicker, so sperm can not enter upper reproductive tract and do not reach ovum. Changes in uterotubal fluid also impair sperm migration. Alteration of the endometrium prevents implantation of fertilized ovum. This IUD has some anovulatory effect (5-15% of treatment cycles; higher in first years)

COST: $300-400 (Average wholesale price $395)
• The ARCH Foundation supplies Mirena intrauterine contraceptives to providers caring for economically disadvantaged women whose insurance does not cover Mirena. They also provide funds for removal to qualifying individuals. Go to www.archfoundation.com
• Mirena units that are contaminated or must be removed in first 3 months or are ◄ expelled *may* be replaced free of cost. Contact Berlex: 1-877-393-9071; Fax: 704-357-0036

ADVANTAGES
Menstrual: Dysmenorrhea generally improves
• Menorrhagia improves (90% less blood loss with LNG IUS; 50% with COCs; 30% with prostaglandin inhibitors). Among 44 menorrhagic women receiving Mirena, only 2 were still menorrhagic at 3 months. At 9 and 12 months 21 of 44 were amenorrheic *[Monteiro-2002]*
• After 3 to 4 months of menstrual irregularities (mostly spotting), Mirena decreases menstrual blood loss more than 70% (97% reduction in blood loss in one study) *[Monteiro-2002]*
• Amenorrhea develops in approximately 20% of users by 1 year and in 60% by 5 years
• Decreased surgery (hysterectomies, endometrial ablation, D & C) for menorrhagia, idiopathic causes of bleeding, leiomyomata or adenomyosis
Sexual/psychological:
• Convenient: permits spontaneous sexual activity. Requires no action at time of intercourse
• Reduced fear of pregnancy can make sex more pleasurable
Cancers, tumors and masses: May have protective effect against endometrial cancer
Other: Extremely effective; as effective or more effective than female sterilization
• May be used as the progestin by women on HRT (off-label)
• *Decreased* risk for ectopic pregnancy (15 times lower than non-contraceptors) ◄
• May reduce occurrence of endometrial polyps in breast cancer patients taking tamoxifen
• Several studies show decreased PID, endometritis and cervicitis in LNG-IUD users ◄

DISADVANTAGES
Menstrual: (Removal for any bleeding problem in first year: 7.6%)
• Number of spotting and bleeding days is significantly higher than normal for first few months and lower than normal after 3 to 6 months of using levonorgestrel intrauterine system
• Amenorrhea (a negative if not explained, a positive for some women if explained well in advance) occurs in about 20% of women at one year of use
• Expulsion: 2.9% in women using Mirena exclusively for contraception; 8.9% to 13.6% in women using Mirena to control heavy bleeding *[Diaz-2000]* *[Monteiro-2002]*

Sexual/psychological: Same as Copper IUD except when spotting and bleeding may interfere with sexual activity

Other:
- Offers no protection against viral STIs ←
- May be expelled (median expulsion rate of 4.8% in 19 studies cited in product monograph)
- Persistent unruptured follicles may cause ovarian cysts; most regress spontaneously
- Headaches, acne, mastalgia during first months (less than 3% of women)
- Brief discomfort after insertion or removal

COMPLICATIONS: See 2004 WHO MEC - Appendix: A1 - A8 **and page 86** ←
- PID risk transiently increased after insertion; ovarian cysts
- Perforation of uterus at time of insertion (less than 1 in 1000)
- Ovarian cysts - usually conservative management adequate

CANDIDATES FOR USE: *Think of Mirena as reversible sterilization*
- Women wanting effective, reversible long-term contraception including women wanting to avoid tubal sterilization. While in place, as effective as laparoscopic tubal sterilization
- Can be used in women with heavy menses, cramps or anemia, or DUB who cannot use Copper IUD
- Menopausal women using ERT, with intact uteri, who are unable to tolerate oral progestins are protected against endometrial carcinoma by using a levonorgestrel intrauterine contraceptive (off-label) *[Raudaskoski, 1995] [Luukkainen, Steroids - 2000]*
- Formal FDA approval is being sought for the use of the LNG IUD to treat menorrhagia

PRESCRIBING PRECAUTIONS: See WHO Precautions in Appendix: A-1 - A-8
- May be used by woman with past history of ectopic pregnancy (WHO:1)

INITIATING METHOD: *Each step should be performed slowly and gently*
- *The one-hand insertion technique is different from current Copper IUDs. Training sessions may be set up by calling 1-866-LNG-IUS1.* See Figure 25.3, pages 97-100
- Usually inserted within 7 days of onset of menses to allow hormone levels to be established prior to ovulation
- If no pregnancy exists, it may be possible to insert at other times of cycle. Have her use a backup contraceptive until next period ←
- Insertion tube is 2 mm wider than for copper intrauterine contraceptives; may rarely need to dilate cervix
- Paracervical block may be required in some patients, especially nulliparous patients
- Counsel in advance to expect menstrual cycle changes, including amenorrhea. Women using the levonorgestrel contraceptive system who received information in advance about possible bleeding changes and amenorrhea were significantly more likely to be highly satisfied with the contraceptive. *[Backman-2002]*
- Advise NSAIDs for post-insertion discomfort. If pain persists, she must return

INSTRUCTIONS FOR PATIENT: Similar to copper intrauterine contraceptive, p. 92

FOLLOW-UP: Same as Copper IUD

PROBLEM MANAGEMENT: Similar to Copper T 380-A; see p. 93-94
- *Perforation:* A study from Israel actually looked at serum LNG levels from an omental Mirena. ← They were higher than POP serum levels. So, theoretically, an abdominal Mirena IUD still provides adequate contraceptive effect until it is removed. Condoms still recommended!

FERTILITY AFTER DISCONTINUATION OF METHOD: Immediate return to baseline fertility

Figure 25.3 How to insert Mirena IUS

Preparation for insertion:

- Confirm that the patient understands the method and alternatives and has signed a consent form

- Administer NSAIDS (preferably 1 hour prior to insertion)

- Examine the patient to establish the size and position of the uterus to detect cervicitis or other genital contraindications and to exclude pregnancy.

- **If indicated**, do a vaginal wet mount, obtain cervical cultures, perform a pregnancy test

- Use aseptic technique during insertion. Sterile gloves not needed. Use sterile gloves when learning to insert this IUD. Then can insert using "no-touch technique"

- Cleanse the cervix and vagina with an antiseptic solution

- Administer paracervical block if needed

- Grasp the upper lip of the cervix with a tenaculum and apply gentle traction to align the cervical canal with the uterine cavity and to stabilize cervix

- Carefully sound the uterus to measure its depth and to check the patency of the cervix. If you encounter cervical stenosis, use dilatation, not force, to overcome resistance

- The uterus should sound to a depth of 6 to 9 cm (some providers use no upper limit, especially if being used for noncontraceptive benefits). Insertion of MIRENA into a uterine cavity less than 6.0 cm by sounding may increase the incidence of expulsion, bleeding, pain, perforation and, possibly, pregnancy. (Actually, there are no data on use of Mirena IUS in women with uterus sounding less than 6.0 cm.)

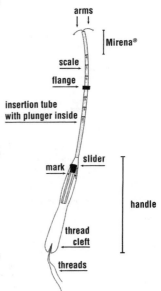

MIRENA® and Inserter

Insertion Procedure:

- Open the sterile package

- Place sterile gloves on your hands or prepare IUS within sterile package

- Pick up the inserter containing MIRENA®

- Carefully release the threads from behind the slider, so that they hang freely

- Make sure that the slider is in the furthest position away from you (positioned at the top of the handle nearest the IUS)

- While looking at the insertion tube, check that the arms of the system are horizontal. If not, align them on a sterile surface or with sterile gloved fingers. This step may be accomplished within sterile package

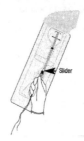

Slider

Checking that the arms of the system are horizontal

- Place the device and the end of the inserter on a sterile surface and pull on both threads to draw the MIRENA® system into the insertion tube (figure a)

- Note that the knobs at the end of the arms now cover the open end of the inserter (figure b)

a) MIRENA® system being drawn into the insertion tube

b) The knobs at the ends of the arms

- Fix the threads in the cleft at end of the handle. If too tight they will not come out and then you will pull the IUD out

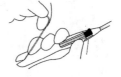

Threads are held in the cleft

- Set the flange to the depth measured by the sound This may be accomplished by placing the insertion tube back into the sterile pack. With the flange in its groove, advance or retract the tubing until the flange is at the cervical position ←

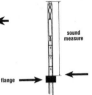

sound measure

flange →

The sound measure

- MIRENA® is now ready to be inserted. Hold the slider firmly in the furthermost position (at the top of the handle). Keep thumb on slider as you insert the inserter. If os is tight and your thumb isn't holding this in place the inserter slides back and the Mirena unloads into the cervix. Grasp the cervix with the tenaculum and apply gentle traction to align the cervical canal with the uterine cavity. Gently insert the inserter into the cervical canal and advance the insertion tube into the uterus until the flange is situated at a distance of about 1.5-2 cm from the external cervical os to give sufficient space for the arms to open. **NOTE: Do not force the inserter**

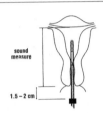

sound measure

1.5 – 2 cm

Flange adjusted to sound depth

- While holding the inserter steady, release the arms of MIRENA® by pulling the slider back until the top of the slider reaches the mark (raised horizontal line on the handle). Wait 30 seconds to allow arms to open ← within the endometrial cavity

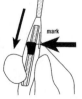

mark

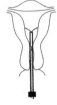

Pulling the slider back to reach the mark   **The arms of the MIRENA® being released**

- Advance the inserter gently toward the fundus until the flange touches the cervix. MIRENA® should now be in the fundal position

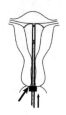

MIRENA® in the fundal position

- Holding the inserter firmly in position release MIRENA® by pulling the slider down all the way. The threads should be released automatically from the cleft. If not released, manually remove the strings from the cleft ◄

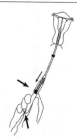

Releasing MIRENA® and withdrawing the inserter

- Remove the inserter from the uterus. Cut the threads to leave about 2 inches (package insert recommends 1.5 to 2.0 cm) visible outside the cervix. **Be sure not to displace the Mirena IUS if cutting the strings with dull scissors. These strings are longer ◄ and tougher than other IUD strings. Give cut strings to patient to feel and to keep**

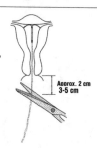

Approx. 2 cm
3-5 cm

Cutting the threads

CHAPTER 26

Combined (Estrogen & Progestin) Contraceptives

www.managingcontraception.com OR www.plannedparenthood.org OR www.noperiod.com

This chapter will describe the methods that provide both an estrogen and a progestin: combined birth control pills (p. 101), the patch (p. 119), then the vaginal ring (p. 121)

PILLS - DAILY "THE PILL" COMBINED PILLS

DESCRIPTION: Each hormonally active pill in combined pills contains an estrogen and a progestin. Ethinyl estradiol
(EE) is the most commonly used estrogen; it is in most 50 μg pills and all of the sub-50 μg formulations. Mestranol, which must be metabolized to EE to become biologically active, is found in two 50 μg formulations (rarely prescribed). At least 7 progestins are used in the different pill formulations. Most packs have 21 active combined pills, with or without 7 additional pills (usually placebo pills). **Monophasic formulations contain active pills with the same amount of hormones in each tablet.** Multiphasic formulations contain active pills with varying amounts of progestin and/or estrogen in the active pills of the cycle. Seasonale has 84 consecutive hormonal pills followed by 7 placebo pills.

EFFECTIVENESS

Perfect use failure rate in first year: 0.3% (of every 1,000 women who take pills for 1 year, 3 will become pregnant in the first year use) (See Table 13.2, p. 39)

Typical use failure rate in first year: 8% *[Trussell J IN Contraceptive Technology, 2004]* ◀
While several studies have found that women in the highest quartile of body weight or highest body mass index (BMI) are at significantly increased risk of OC failure *[Holt-2002] [Holt-2005][Norris-2003]*, other research does not indicate that clinicians need change their prescribing habits for overweight woman *[Vessey-2001][Kaunitz-2002]*. Until there are more ◀ conclusive data an approach might be to avoid the lowest dose combined pills for markedly overweight women.

MECHANISM: Suppresses ovulation (90% to 95% of time). Also causes thickening of cervical mucus, which blocks sperm penetration and entry into the upper reproductive tract. Thin, asynchronous endometrium inhibits implantation. Tubal motility slowed.

COST

- Cost of one cycle: from a few dollars to more than $50. Most pharmacies charge $20-$42/cycle
- Costs differ from region to region, and pills with 50 mcg of estrogen often cost more.
- Generic brands are generally less expensive. They are not required to have clinical testing; they must only prove blood level equivalency (80–125% of parent compound's blood levels).
- Most major insurance companies cover at least some brands of pills
- The co-pay for Seasonale is increased to as much as $60 per a package that covers a ◀ woman for 3 months

ADVANTAGES

Menstrual:
- Decreased blood loss and decreased anemia may decrease menstrual cramps/pain, and more predictable menses
- Eliminates ovulation pain (Mittelschmerz)
- Can be used to manipulate timing and frequency of menses (see Choice of COC, p. 110 & 115)

- Reduces risk of internal hemorrhage from ovulation (especially important in women with bleeding diatheses or women using anticoagulants)
- Regulates menses and provides progestin for women with anovulation/PCOS (reducing risk of endometrial cancer)

Sexual/psychological:
- No interruption at time of intercourse; more spontaneous activity
- Intercourse may be more pleasurable because of reduced risk of pregnancy

Cancers/tumors/masses:
- Low dose OCs offer the same 50% reduction in ovarian cancer risk as higher-dose formulations *[Ness-2000]*. COC users for 5 years have 50% reduction in risk; users for 10 years have 80% reduction. Protection extends for 30 years beyond last pill use; Significant reduction in risk also seen in some high risk women carrying BRCA mutations
- Decreased risk for **endometrial cancer** *[Grimes-2001]* (30 µg and higher dose pills)
  - COC users for 1 year have 20% reduction in risk; users for 4 years have 60% reduction
  - Protection extends for 30 years beyond last pill use *[Ness, AmJEpidemiol-2000]*
  - Particularly important for PCOS women, obese women, and perimenopausal women
- Decreased risk of death from **colorectal cancer** *[Beral-1999]*
- Decreased risk of corpus luteum cysts and hemorrhagic corpus luteum cysts
- *Breast masses:* 25% reduction in all **benign breast disease** (including fibroadenomas)

DO BIRTH CONTROL PILLS CAUSE BREAST CANCER?

- After more than 50 studies, most experts believe *that pills have little, if any, effect on the risk of developing breast cancer.*
- The Women's Care Study of 4575 women with breast cancer and 4682 controls found no increased risk for breast cancer (RR: 1.0) among women currently using pills and a decreased risk of breast cancer (RR: 0.9) for those women who had previously used pills. Use of pills by women with a family history of breast cancer was not associated with an increased risk of breast cancer, nor was the initiation of pill use at a young age *[Marchbanks - 2002]*
- However, several studies have shown that current users of pills are slightly more likely to be **diagnosed** with breast cancer (Relative Risk: 1.2). *[Collaborative Group; Lancet 1996]*
- Two factors may explain the increased risk of breast cancer being diagnosed in women currently taking pills: 1) a **detection bias** (more breast exams and more mammography) or 2) **promotion** of an already present nidus of cancer cells
- Ten years after discontinuing pills, women who have taken pills are at no increased risk for having breast cancer diagnosed. *[Collaborative Group; Lancet 1996]*
- Breast cancers diagnosed in women currently on pills or women who have taken pills in the past are more likely to be localized *(less likely to be metastatic)*. *[Collaborative Group; Lancet 1996]*
- By the age of 55, the risk of having had breast cancer diagnosed is the same for women who have used pills and those who have not
- The conclusion of the largest collaborative study of the risk for breast cancer is that women with a strong family Hx of breast cancer do not further increase their risk for breast cancer risk by taking pills. *[Collaborative Group; Lancet 1996]* This was also the conclusion of the Nurses Health Study *[Lipnick-1986] [Colditz-1996]* and the Cancer and Steroid Hormone (CASH) study. *[Murray-1989] [The Centers for Disease Control Cancer and Steroid Hormone Study-1983]*
- While there are still unanswered questions about pills and breast cancer, today, four decades after their arrival on the contraceptive scene, the overall conclusion is that pills do not cause breast cancer. *"Many years after stopping oral contraceptive use, the main effect may be protection against metastatic disease."* *[Speroff and Darney-2001] [Collaborative Group; Lancet 1996]*

NOTE: Many of the symptoms women complain of after starting pills (nausea, headaches, bloating) occur more frequently during the days a woman is on placebo pills. Therefore, ask women *when* they have these symptoms. **Symptoms occurring primarily during the placebo days may be an indication for extended or continuous use of pills** *[Sulak-2002]*
Other:

- Reduces risk of ectopic pregnancy and risk of hospitalization with diagnosis of PID
- Treatment for acne, hirsutism and other androgen excess/sensitivity states
- Reduced vasomotor symptoms and effective contraception in perimenopausal women
- Increased bone mineral density. Pills with 35 micrograms of estrogen used by women in their 40s; have been associated with fewer postmenopausal hip fractures *[Michaelsson-1998; Lancet, 353:1481-1484]*. 20-30 mcg EE likely to have similar benefit
- Decreased pain and frequency of sickle cell disease crises

DISADVANTAGES

Menstrual:

- Spotting, particularly during first few cycles and with inconsistent use
- Scant or missed menses possible, not clinically significant but can cause worry
- Post-pill amenorrhea (lasts up to 6 months). Uncommon and usually in women with history of irregular periods prior to taking pills

Sexual/psychological:

- Decreased libido and anorgasmias are possible, but unusual. It is unknown why. The effects of COCs on anorgasmias are unlikely to be testosterone related
- Mood changes, depression, anxiety, irritability, fatigue may develop while on COCs, but no more frequent than with placebos. Rule out other causes before implicating COCs
- Daily pill taking may be stressful (especially if privacy is an issue)

Cancers/tumors/masses: **Breast cancer** - see comprehensive answer on previous page
- *Cervical cancer:*
  - No consistent increased risk seen for squamous cell cervical carcinoma (85% of all cervical cancer) after controlling for confounding variables, such as number of sex partners
  - Risk of a relatively uncommon type of cervical cancer, adenocarcinoma, is increased 60%, but no extra screening required other than recommended Pap screening
- *Hepatocellular adenoma:* risk increased among COC users (only ≥ 50 μg formulations). Risk of hepatic carcinoma not increased, even in populations with high prevalence of hepatitis B

Other:

- No protection against STIs, including HIV.
- Shedding of HIV may be slightly increased
- Not recommened with use of some antiretrovirals
- Nausea or vomiting, especially in first few cycles
- Breast tenderness or pain
- Headaches: may increase
- Increased varicosities, chloasma, spiders
- Daily dosing is difficult for some women

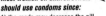

Most women on antiretrovirals should use condoms since:
1) the meds may decrease the pill effectiveness if the antiretroviral induces cytochrome p 450 metabolism
2) GI side-effects from drugs may decrease OC effectiveness

- Average weight gain no different among COC users than in placebo users (see NOTE below). There is no evidence that pills are implicated in the U.S. "obesity epidemic" ◀━
- See COMPLICATIONS section below

NOTE: Medical problems and abnormal symptom complaints are frequently attributed by patients and providers to COC use. While some women may be particularly sensitive to sex steroids, a recent placebo-controlled study found that the incidence of all of the frequently mentioned hormone-related side effects was not significantly different in the COC group than it was in the placebo group *[Redmond, 1999]* For example, headaches occurred in 18.4% of women on Ortho Tricyclen and in 20.5% of women in the placebo group. Nausea occurred in 12.7% of women on Ortho Tricyclen and in 9.0 % of women on placebo pills. Weight gain occurred in 2.2% of women on Ortho Tricyclen and in 2.1 % of women on placebo pills

COMPLICATIONS

- *Venous thromboembolism (VTE)*
  - The risk of VTE with COC use is less than with pregnancy:

No COC use	4-8/100,000 women per year
COC use	10-30/100,000 women per year
Pregnancy	60/100,000 women per year

  - DVT risk is associated with the dose of estrogen; the risk of VTE in 50 μg pills is greater than in 20-35 μg pills. The type of progestin may *slightly* influence DVT risk; If true, this risk is still only one-half the VTE risk associated with pregnancy. The current labeling for desogestrel pills states that "several epidemiologic studies indicate that third generation oral contraceptives, including those containing desogestrel, are associated with a higher risk of venous thromboembolism than certain second generations OCs. In general, these studies indicate an approximate 2-fold increased risk, which corresponds to an additional 1-2 cases of venous thromboembolism per 10,000 women-years of use. However, data from additional studies have not shown this 2-fold increase in risk." Neither the U.S. Food & Drug Administration (FDA) nor the American College of Obstetricians (ACOG) recommends switching current users of desogestrel containing pills to other products. Underlying blood dyscrasias such as Factor V_{Leiden} mutation and Protein S or C abnormalities increase risk of VTE significantly. However, in the absence of strong family history (see boxed message on p. 98), screening is not necessary. Yasmin, the newest OC formulation, probably has intial DVT rates in line with all other OCs
- *Myocardial infarction (MI) and stroke*
  - There is no increased risk of MI or stroke for young women who are using low-dose COCs who do not smoke, do not have hypertension and do not have migraine headaches with neurological findings
  - Women at risk:
    - Smokers over 35 shouldn't use COCs; all smokers should be encouraged to stop smoking. Smokers over 35 have MI rate of 396 per million COC users per year vs. 88 per million non-COC users per year
    - Women with hypertension, diabetes, hyperlipidemia or obesity
    - Women with migraine with aura (only stroke risk increases)
- *Hypertension:* 1% of users develop hypertension which (usually) is reversible within 1-3 months of discontinuing COCs. Most users have a very small increase if any in blood pressure

---

ELEVATED BLOOD PRESSURE: A TEACHABLE MOMENT

Each time you find an elevated blood pressure, several messages. should reach the ears of your patient*:

1. If you smoke, stop smoking. This is by far the most important step you can take
2. Moderate exercise for 20-30 minutes each day, every day reduces blood pressure!
3. If overweight, lose weight. Reduce fat in your diet
4. Use salt in moderation
5. If you are on antihypertensive medications, take them regularly!
6. Work on reducing stress in your life (may be difficult and may take time)

* In addition to deciding if pills can be used ←

- *Neoplasia:* COC users using early high dose pills are at higher risk of developing adenocarcinoma (rare) of the cervix and hepatic adenomas (rare). See boxed message on p. 94 for an answer to the question: Do birth control pills cause breast cancer?
- *Cholelithiasis/cholecystitis:* higher dose formulations were associated with increased risk of symptomatic gallbladder disease
  - Sub-50 mcg formulations may be neutral or have a slightly increased risk
  - Use COCs with caution in women with known gallstones. Asymptomatic (WHO:2), treated by cholecystectomy (WHO:2), symptomatic and being treated medically (WHO:3), current and symptomatic (WHO:3)
- *Visual changes:* Rare cases of retinal thrombosis (must stop pills). Contact lens users may have dry eye. May need to recommend eye drops or need to switch methods

CANDIDATES FOR USE: See 2004 WHO Medical Eligibility Criteria, p. A-1 through A-8

- Most healthy reproductive aged women are candidates for COCs
- For healthy women, the use of COCs is often decided on the basis of a balance of perceived benefits and side effects
- In addition to medical precautions, real world considerations such as the need for privacy, affordable access to COCs, and the requirement for daily administration need to be considered when evaluating a woman for COC use

Adolescents

  - May be excellent candidates for contraceptive benefits if patient is able to take a pill each day.
  - Many of the non-contraceptive effects of OCs are particularly important for adolescent women – e.g. decreased dysmenorrhea (the most common cause of lost days of school and work among women under 25), and decreased acne, hirsutism, or hypoestrogenism due to eating disorders, excessive exercise, stress, etc.
  - Failure rates are higher in teens using COCs. Help teens integrate pill taking into daily rituals (tooth brushing, beeper, watch alarm, application of makeup, putting on earrings). Ask teenager how she will create a way to be successful. Ask if parents are aware that she is using contraception and if they are supportive. Consider continuous COC use. See p. 107
  - If at risk for STIs, encourage teens to use condoms consistently and correctly
  - Be sure she has a package of Plan B (levonorgestrel ECPs) at home

SPECIAL CONSIDERATIONS FOR USE

- Women with medical conditions that improve with COCs may find COCs a particularly attractive contraceptive option. This includes women with endometriosis, menstrual migraine (in some instances), iron deficiency anemia, acne, hirsutism, polycystic ovarian syndrome (PCOS), ovarian or endometrial cancer risk factors, eating disorders or activity patterns that increase risk of osteoporosis. Consider continuous or extended COC use with Seasonale or another monophasic pill. See p. 107
- Women whose reproductive health would be improved by ovulation suppression or decreased menstrual blood loss should also consider COCs. This includes women with chronic amenorrhea (unopposed estrogen), and women who suffer menorrhagia or dysmenorrhea and some anticoagulated women (COCs decrease risk of internal hemorrhage with ovulation and menorrhagia) and women using seizure medication (decrease menorrhagia)
- Women whose quality of life would be improved by reducing frequency of or eliminating menses with extended cycles or continuous COC use: See next page

- Women who have difficulty swallowing pills may benefit from the chewable formulation of Ovcon-35. Also, pills carried about may be taken at any time without water, potentially leading to fewer missed pills and greater privacy. OCs may also be placed in the vagina ◄ for systemic absorption

PRESCRIBING PRECAUTIONS

See WHO Eligibility Criteria Appendix A1 - A8

- Thrombophlebitis, thromboembolic disease or history of deep venous thrombosis or pulmonary embolism (unless anticoagulated)
- Family history of close family members with unexplained VTE at early age (eg Factor V_{Leiden} mutation)

The questions to ask are as follows:

- Has a close family member (parents, siblings, grandparents, uncles, aunts) ever had unexplained blood clots in the legs or lungs?
- Has a close family member ever been hospitalized for blood clots in the legs or lungs? If so, did this person take a blood thinner? (If not, it is likely that the family member had a nonsignificant condition such as superficial phlebitis or varicose veins)
- What were the circumstances in which the blood clot took place (eg. cancer, airline travel, surgery, obesity, immobility, postpartum, etc.)? *[Grimes - 1999]*

"If the family history screening is positive - one or more close family members with a definite strong VTE history (young first - or second - degree relatives with spontaneous VTE) clinician might consider further laboratory screening for genetic conditions. Another alternative is to suggest progestin-only OCs or another non-estrogen-containing birth control method." *[Grimes - 1999]*

- Cerebral vascular disease or coronary artery disease
- Current breast cancer (WHO: 4)
- Past breast cancer and no evidence of current disease for 5 years (WHO: 3)
- Endometrial carcinoma or other estrogen dependent neoplasia (excluding endometriosis and leiomyoma) WHO rates endometrial cancer a "1" for COCs
- Unexplained vaginal bleeding suspicious for serious condition (before evaluation) (WHO: 2)
- Cholestatic jaundice of pregnancy or jaundice with prior pill use
- Hepatic adenoma or carcinoma or significant hepatic dysfunction
- Smoking after age 35. WHO defines heavy smoking as $\geq$ 15 cigarettes/day (see p. A3)
- Complicated or prolonged diabetes, systemic lupus erythematosus (if vascular changes)
- Severe migraine with aura or other neurologic symptoms
- Breastfeeding women (without supplementation) until breastfeeding well established COCs have no adverse effects on babies of OC-using, nursing mothers ◄
- Hypersensitivity to any components of pills
- Daily use of certain broadspectrum antibiotics. Although WHO (see p. A8) states that women using antibiotics other than grisiofulvin or rifampicin may use COCs (WHO:1), patients are exposed to conflicting information. Many clinicians explain the differing opinons and let patient decide for herself. There are not convincing data that broad specrum antibiotics increase the failure of COCs. Doxycycline and tetracycline do not ◄ lower the effectiveness of COCs *(Murphy AA, 1991) (Neely JL, 1991)*
- Hypertension with vascular disease $\dfrac{140\text{-}159}{90\text{-}99}$ = 3 (WHO) $\dfrac{\geq 160}{\geq 100}$ = 4 (WHO)

EXTENDED USE OF PILLS MAY MEAN:

A. Manipulation of a cycle to delay one period for a trip, honeymoon, or athletic event

B. Use of active hormonal pills for more than 21 consecutive days) followed by 2 to 7 hormone-free days. Seasonale is a COC packaged to produce 4 cycles per year. The hormones in Seasonale ARE THE SAME 30 mcg EE pills with levonorgestrel: Nordette, Lo-Oval, etc. Pills other than Seasonale may be used to accomplish this same end.

C. Continuous daily COCs for at least 21 pills, but after that, may break for 2-7 days if spotting or breakthrough bleeding is bothersome

D. Use of a monophasic pill indefinitely. BTB can occur at any time with this regimen. Eventually she develops an atrophic endometrium and breakthrough bleeding decreases

Cyclic symptoms that may improve from the extended use of pills:

Symptoms usually occurring at the time of menses: (predicted benefits)

- Abdominal, back or leg pain, dysmenorrhea, endometriosis Sx *[Vercellini-2003]*
- Bleeding abnormalities including menorrhagia
- Irritability or depression. Decreased libido
- Headaches including both menstrual migraine and other cyclic headaches *[Sulak-2000] [Kwiecien-2003]*
- Nausea, dizziness, vomiting or diarrhea
- Cyclic yeast or other infections or cyclic nosebleeds
- Cyclic seizures, arthritis, or recurrences of asthma at the time of menses
- Changes in insulin requirements
- Cyclic symptoms associated with polycystic ovarian disease

Symptoms usually occurring at midcycle:(predicted benefits)

- Spotting due to sudden fall in estradiol
- Sharp or dull pain (that precedes ovulation and is caused by high midcycle PG levels)

Symptoms usually occurring just prior to menses: (predicted benefits)

- Slight to more dramatic weight gain, bloating, swollen eyes or ankles
- Breast fullness or tenderness
- Anxiety, irritability or depression, nausea or headaches due to dropping estrogen
- Acne, spotting, discharge, breast fullness or tenderness
- Pain or cramping or constipation

Most important advantages & disadvantages of taking COCs continuously:

Advantages:

- May be more effective as a contraceptive when taken daily
- May be easier to remember (do the same thing every day)
- Women wanting to avoid bleeding for an athletic event, special trip or any other reason
- Less frequent menstruation *[Sulak-2000] [Glasier-2003]* and less blood loss
- Decreased expenses from tampons, pads, pain meds, and days of work missed ←

Disadvantages:

- More expensive and the extra packs of pills required may not be covered by insurance
- Unscheduled spotting or bleeding and the absence of regular menses

- Clinician must explain that amenorrhea, while taking a progestin every day, is not ← harmful. While ammenorhea for a woman on no hormonal contraceptive, may lead to endometrial hyperplasia or cancer.

MEDICAL ELIGIBILITY CHECKLIST: Ask a woman on pills the questions below. If she answers NO to ALL of the questions and has no other contraindications, then she can use low-dose COCs if she wants. If she answers YES to a question below, follow the instructions

1. Do you think you are pregnant?

☐ No ☐ Yes   Assess if pregnant. If she might be pregnant, give her male or female condoms to use until reasonably certain that she is not pregnant. Then she can start COCs. If unprotected sex within past 5 days, consider emergency contraception if she is not pregnant

2. Do you smoke cigarettes and are you age 35 or older?

☐ No ☐ Yes   Urge her to stop smoking. If she is 35 or older and she will not stop smoking, do not provide COCs. Help her choose a method without estrogen

3. Do you have high blood pressure? (see Appendix, p. A2)

☐ No ☐ Yes   If BP below 140/90, OK to give COCs if no other comorbidities exist even if taking antihypertensive drugs. If BP is elevated, see Appendix, p. A-3. Consider IUD or progestin-only methods

4. Are you breast-feeding your baby?

☐ No ☐ Yes   No controversy: Provide interval contraceptive she may use while nursing. Provide COCs and counsel to start when she adds nutrition from other sources (formula or solid foods). Give her ECPs and condom. May start COCs after lactation well established.

5. Do you have serious medical problems such as a heart disease, severe chest pain, blood clots, high blood pressure or diabetes? Have you ever had such problems?

☐ No ☐ Yes   Do not provide COCs if she reports heart attack or heart disease due to blocked arteries, stroke, blood clots (except superficial clots), severe chest pain with unusual shortness of breath, diabetes for more than 20 years, or damage to vision, kidneys, or nervous system caused by diabetes. Help her choose a method without estrogen. Consider POPs, LNg IUD, Copper T 380 A, Implanon, barriers, DMPA

6. Do you have or have you ever had breast cancer? (see p. A4)

☐ No ☐ Yes   Do not provide COCs if current or less than 5 years ago. Help her choose a method without hormones. If disease free x 5 years, may consider COCs (WHO: 3)

7. Do you often get bad headaches with blurred vision, nausea or dizziness?

☐ No ☐ Yes   If she gets migraine headaches with blurred vision, temporary loss of vision, sees flashing lights or zigzag lines, or trouble speaking or moving, or has other neurologic symptoms, do not provide COCs. Consider POPs, LNG IUD, Copper T 380 A, Implanon, barriers. Help her choose a method without estrogen. If she has only menstrual migraines without abnormal neurologic findings, consider COC use.

8. Are you taking medicine for seizures or are you taking rifampin, griseofulvin or St. John's Wort?

☐ No ☐ Yes   If she is using St. John's Wort, rifampin, griseofulvin, topiramate (Topomax) phenytoin, carbamazepine, barbiturates, or primidone, guide her to DMPA or a non-hormonal method or strongly encourage condom use as backup contraceptive. Use of valproic acid does NOT lower the effectiveness of COCs. See discussion p. 107

9. Do you have vaginal bleeding that is unusual for you? (see Appendix, p. A3)

☐ No ☐ Yes   If she is not likely to be pregnant but has unexplained vaginal bleeding that suggests an underlying medical condition, evaluate condition before initiating pills. Treat as appropriate or refer. Reassess COC use based on findings

10. Do you have jaundice, cirrhosis of the liver, an acute liver infection or tumor? (Are her eyes or skin unusually yellow?) (see p. A5)

☐ No ☐ Yes   If she has serious active liver disease (jaundice, painful or enlarged liver, active viral hepatitis, liver tumor), do not provide COCs. Refer for care as appropriate. Help her choose a method without hormones

11. Do you have gallbladder disease? Ever had jaundice while taking COCs or during pregnancy?

☐ No ☐ Yes   If she has acute gallbladder disease now or takes medicine for gallbladder disease, or if she has had jaundice while using COCs or during pregnancy, do not provide COCs. Consider a method without estrogen. Women with known asymptomatic cholelithiasis may use COCs with caution

12. Are you planning surgery with a recovery period that will keep you from walking for a week or more? Have you had a baby in the past 21 days?

☐ No ☐ Yes   Help her choose a method without estrogen. If planning surgery or just had a baby, provide COCs for delayed initiation and another interim method

13. Have you ever become pregnant on the pill?

☐ No ☐ Yes   Ask about pill-taking habits. Consider longer dosing hormonal methods or shortening or eliminating the pill-free interval while using COCs

INITIATING METHOD (see INSTRUCTIONS FOR PATIENT, p. 111)
- In asymptomatic women, **a pelvic examination is not necessary to start pills** *[Stewart-2001]*
- *Counseling is critical in helping women successfully use the pill*
  - Patients who are counseled well about how to use pills and what side effects may develop are usually better prepared and may be more likely to continue use
- *Timing of initiation* (see Table 26.2, p. 114)
  - First day of next menstrual period start. **"Quick Start"** (starting the day of the counseling ◄ clinic visit) is quite feasible to help women adapt to COCs *[Westoff-2002]*. Provide 7 day backup. Bleeding is not increased in "quick starters". This is now the preferred method of starting pills
  - If using Sunday start, recommend back-up method x 7 days. Sunday start can result in no periods on weekends
- *Choice of pill*
  - The pill that will work best for the woman is the one that she will take regularly
  - For special situations, some formulations offer advantages over others (see CHOOSING COCs FOR WOMEN IN SPECIAL SITUATIONS, next page)
    - In general, use the lowest dose of hormones that will provide pregnancy protection, deliver the non-contraceptive benefits that are important to the woman, and minimize her side effects

- Monophasic formulations are preferable if women are interested in controlling cycle lengths or timing by eliminating any or all pill-free intervals for medical indications or personal preference (see Choosing COCs, Figure 26.2 p. 115)
- Triphasic formulations may be preferable to use to reduce some side effects (such as premenstrual breakthrough bleeding) when it is not desirable to increase hormone levels throughout the entire cycle or when it is desirable to reduce total cycle progestin levels (e.g. acne treatment). There are no studies showing the superiority ← of triphasic pills for women with BTB
- *Choice of pattern of COC use*
  - 28-day cycling: Most common use pattern. Women have monthly withdrawal bleeding during placebo pills
  - *"First day start" each cycle:* Women can start each new pack of pills on first day of menses each cycle
  - *"Bicycling" or "tricycling":* Women skip placebo pills for either 1 or 2 packs and then use the placebo pills and have withdrawal bleeding every 7 weeks (end of 2nd pack) or 10 weeks (end of 3rd pack). **Use monophasic pills**
  - You may prescribe 4 packs of low dose monophasic pills omitting the placebo pills. The new pill, *Seasonale*, is packaged to provide pills in this manner: 84 active pills followed by 7 days of inactive pills, resulting in 4 withdrawal bleeds/year
  - *"Continuous use":* Women take only active pills and have no withdrawal bleeding. Often women must transition through bicycling or tricycling to achieve amenorrhea. Must use monophasic pills. Need to counsel regarding BTB and spotting
  - *NOTE: the last three options may be particularly good for:*
    - Women with menstrually-related problems (menorrhagia, anemia, dysmenorrhea, menstrual mood changes, menstrual irregularity, endometriosis, menstrual migraine, PMS, PMDD)
    - Women on medications that reduce COC effectiveness (e.g. anticonvulsants, St. John's Wort)
    - Women who have conceived while on COCs or who forget to take them regularly
    - Women who are ambulatory but disabled and for whom menstrual bleeding may be particularly problematic
    - Women who want to control their cycles for their own convenience

CHOOSING COCs FOR WOMEN IN SPECIAL SITUATIONS

- *Endometriosis:* Seasonale and other pills taken continuously are most effective in reducing symptoms. Continuous use (no break) of ring may also be effective
- *Functional ovarian cysts:* higher dose monophasic COCs may be slightly more effective. Extended or continuous use of pills may also be more effective
- *Androgen excess states:* all COCs with higher estrogen/progestin ratios are preferable to reduce free testosterone and inhibit 5 alpha-reductase activity.
- *Breastfeeding women:* progestin-only methods preferable to COCs in breastfeeding women. COCs may be considered when baby's diet supplemented by other sources of nutrition or after lactation well established (if patient prefers COCs)

- *Hypercholesterolemia:* Selection of pill depends on type of dyslipidemia:
  - Elevated LDL or low HDL: consider estrogenic pill (high estrogen/androgen rates)
  - Elevated triglycerides: Some clinicians recommend not prescribing COCs if triglycerides > 350 mg/dL because COCs increase triglycerides by approximately 30% and risk of pancreatitis increased (norgestimate may increase triglycerides less)
- *Hepatic enzyme-inducing agents (e.g. anticonvulsants except valproic acid and St. John's Wort):* Options:
  - Prescribe high-dose COC (containing 50 µg EE)
  - Prescribe 30-35 µg pill with reduced pill-free interval (first-day start, bicycling with first day start, or continuous use)
- *Antibiotic use:* Concern that without intestinal flora to unconjugate the hormonal compounds produced by first hepatic processing, subsequent reabsorption of estrogen and progestin would not be possible. However, research on current dose pills suggests no significant difference in circulating serum levels of hormones when women used broad-spectrum antibiotics *(Murphy AA-1991)(Neely-1991)*. Class OC labeling warns about potential antibiotic ◄ interactions. If patient has other risk factor (vomiting, diarrhea, forgetfulness) or is worried, ◄ do suggest back-up method for duration of antibiotic use. Rifampin **does** and griseofulvin **may** decrease pill effectiveness and a backup or alternative contraceptive is recommended. Check PDR for effects of antiretrovirals on steroid levels. Antiretrovirals receive a 2 ◄ (generally use the method) in the WHO Medical Eligibility Criteria
- *Obese patients:* Current data do not suggest different prescribing for markedly ◄— overweight women

INSTRUCTIONS FOR PATIENT: Periodic "breaks" from pills are NOT recommended!

- Key to successful pill use is a well-informed patient. Provide new-start patients with:
  - Clear instructions on pill initiation, preferably written and in her primary language. If reasonably certain that she is not pregnant, use Quick Start technique *[Westhoff - 2002]* *(See p. 105).* Have her take the first hormonally active pill immediately and use all pills. This *may* delay onset of next period. This will not increase the number of days of menstrual bleeding nor the number of days of spotting. The 3 month continuation rate among Quick Start women was markedly better than women starting pills at later times
  - Help her plan where to store pills, how to remember to take them and where to obtain refills
  - Explanation about possible transitional side effects (spotting, breast tenderness, headaches, etc.) and encouragement to call or return should any become troublesome (see PROBLEM MANAGEMENT). Also highlight noncontraceptive benefits
  - Warning about serious complications (see ACHES, p. A-29)
- Backup method: ensure patient has and knows how to use method if she needs to use one for interim protection, back-up, or as an alternate method if she ever discontinues COC use.
- Have patient return in 3 months for BP check and follow-up of any complaints (there ◄— is some debate about this recommendation especially if a woman can get the blood pressure determination elsewhere). Subsequently, only annual routine gynecologic exams are offered to low-risk patients
- Each woman on birth control pills needs a package of Plan B in her medicine chest ◄—

Before you are seen by a counselor or clinician, please tell us your response to the following questions. Please check yes or no. Tell us if you have:

Any problem you think could be caused by pills	Yes_____	No_____
Nausea or vomiting	Yes_____	No_____
Spotting or irregular vaginal bleeding	Yes_____	No_____
Occasional missed periods (no bleeding)	Yes_____	No_____
Breast tenderness or a breast lump	Yes_____	No_____
Any symptoms of pregnancy	Yes_____	No_____
Depression, severe anxiety or mood changes	Yes_____	No_____
Decreased interest in sex	Yes_____	No_____
Decreased ability to have orgasms	Yes_____	No_____
Gained 5 pounds or more	Yes_____	No_____
High blood pressure	Yes_____	No_____
Been smoking at all	Yes_____	No_____
Been taking medicines for seizures	Yes_____	No_____
Been taking over-the-counter herbs	Yes_____	No_____
Ever forgotten to take your pills	Yes_____	No_____
Forgotten to take pills quite often	Yes_____	No_____
Changed sexual partners	Yes_____	No_____

Experienced any of the following pill danger signals:

__A__bdominal pain?	Yes_____	No_____
Yellow skin or eyes?	Yes_____	No_____
__C__hest pain?	Yes_____	No_____
__H__eadaches which are severe?	Yes_____	No_____
__E__ye problems: blurred vision or loss of vision?	Yes_____	No_____
__S__evere leg pain?	Yes_____	No_____

"**ACHES**" is a way for you to remember the pill danger signals.
Please explain __any__ question you have answered "yes" to:

PROBLEM MANAGEMENT

Nausea/vomiting: **Rule out pregnancy, reassure that nausea usually improves**

- Prescribe lower estrogen formulation
- Suggest taking pills at night (evening meal or bedtime) to allow patient to sleep through high serum levels of hormones. Suggest taking pills with morning meal if experiencing bothersome nausea during the night
- If patient vomits within one hour of taking pill, suggest antiemetic prior to taking replacement pill. Use backup method for 7 days
- Consider change to a non-oral route of delivery (IUD or ring) ◄
- Abdominal pain problems possibly related to COCs: thrombosis of major intra-abdominal vessels, gallstones, pancreatitis, liver adenoma, Crohn's disease or porphyria

Spotting and/or breakthrough bleeding:

- See Fig. 26.3, p. 116 for women taking pills in the traditional 21/7 manner.

Women taking pills for an extended period of time: ◄

- Take first 21 pills every single day whether or not spotting occurs
- Thereafter, one approach to spotting is to stop active hormonal pills on first day of spotting (after having taken pills for at least 21 days). Take no pill for 2 or 3 days. Then restart pills daily until the next spotting day (again as long as pill has been ◄ taken for at least 21 days). Days of spotting taking pills continuously will decrease over time as occurs with all pills

Missed one pill: **Instruct patient to take missed pill ASAP and take next pill as usual**

- Offer emergency contraceptive pills (ECPs), especially if missed pill is at beginning of pack.

Missed two pills:

- Instruct patient to take one of the forgotten pills every 12 hours until she gets caught up, then continue rest of pack. Backup contraception recommended for 7 days
- Additionally, offer ECPs, especially if patient is early in cycle and continue COCs next day

Missed more than two pills: **Offer ECPs. Actually, provide ECPs in advance**

- If she had intercourse, have her take EC and restart OCs the next day. Use barrier for 7 days
- If patient declines ECPs, instruct patient to skip missed pills and complete rest of pills in pack, but to use barrier method with each act of intercourse until her next menses. Advise patient that pills may not provide protection, but will help control her cycle

If patient uses ECPs:

- Instruct patient to resume taking pills in pack the next day after she finishes ECPs

Missed withdrawal bleed on COCs (not on extended or continuous cycles):

- Offer pregnancy test, especially if she missed any pills in last cycle or if she has any symptoms of pregnancy
- Offer emergency contraception if any recent unprotected intercourse
- Advise patient that there are no adverse clinical impacts of amenorrhea from COCs
- If patient prefers monthly withdrawal bleeding, consider switching to formulation with higher estrogen or lower progestin
- Otherwise, have her continue her COCs on usual schedule

New onset or significant worsening of headaches on COCs: (see Figure 26.4, p. 117)

Hot flashes on placebo-pill week:

- Suggest starting on first day of withdrawal bleeding or continuous use of monophasic pills OR
- Offer low-dose of transdermal or oral estrogen during placebo-pill week

MAKING THE TRANSITION FROM COCs TO HRT: (See Figure 26.5, p. 118)

FERTILITY AFTER DISCONTINUATION OF METHOD

- Immediate return of fertility: Average delay in ovulation 1-2 weeks. Post-pill amenorrhea more common in women with a past history of very irregular menses; rarely persists for up to 6 months
- Women should initiate another method immediately after discontinuing COCs
- Women should be advised that their pattern of menses **prior** to starting pills (frequency, duration, flow, dysmenorrhea) **tends to return** once they stop COCs
- Taking pills for 5-10 years prior to trying to become pregnant may actually protect a woman from some of the causes of infertility such as endometriosis, endometrial cancer, uterine fibroids, polycystic ovarian disease and ovarian cancer

Table 26.2 Starting Combined Oral Contraceptives*

CONDITION BEFORE STARTING	WHEN TO START COCs?
Starting (restarting) COCs in menstruating women	• Immediately, if pregnancy excluded start with first pill in package; backup needed x 7 days "QUICK START" *[Westoff - 2002]* See p. 109 • First day of next menses • Within 5 days after start of her menstrual bleeding**. • First Sunday after next menses begins**. Backup needed x 7 days
Starting (restarting) in amenorrheic women	Anytime if it is reasonably certain that she is not pregnant; abstain from sex or use backup method for next 7 days
Postpartum and breast-feeding	If still breastfeeding & less than 6 months PP, wait at least until the baby is receiving significant nutritional supplement If more than 6 months PP & amenorrheic, start COCs as advised for other amenorrheic woman
Postpartum and not breast-feeding (after pregnancy of 24 or more weeks)	• Wait 3 weeks after delivery to allow hypercoagulable state of pregnancy to abate
After 1st or 2nd trimester (≤ 24 weeks) pregnancy loss or termination	• Immediately - start the same day No backup needed
Switching from another hormonal method	• Start COCs immediately if she has been using hormonal method correctly and consistently, or if it is reasonably certain she is not pregnant. No need to wait until next period. No additional contraceptive needed • If previous method was an injectable, start COCs at the time repeat injection would have been given
Switching from a non-hormonal method (other than IUD)	• Can start immediately or at any other time if it is reasonably certain that she is not pregnant. Use backup method for the next 7 days unless it is the first day of menses
Switching from an IUD (including hormonal)	• Start pills within 5 days of start of mentrual bleeding, no additional contraceptive needed & IUD can be removed at that time • Start pills at any other time if it is reasonably certain she is not pregnant. If sexually active in this menstrual cycle and more than 5 days since menstrual bleeding started, remove IUD at time of next menstrual period OR give EC, then start COCs immediately; backup x 7 days
After taking ECPs	• Day after ECP** • First day of next menses** } if using other interim • Sunday of next menses** } method until menses

* World Health Organization. Selected Practice Recommendations for Contraceptive Use. 2004
** Back-up method needed for 7 days after starting COCs if it has been more than 5 days since menstrual bleeding started

Figure 26.2

CHOOSING A PILL

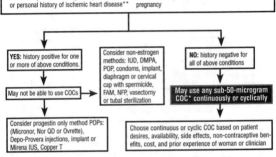

Woman wants to use "the Pill"
Does she have problem of:
- Smoking & age 35 or older
- Hypertension (See appendix, A-3)
- Undiagnosed abnormal vaginal bleeding
- Diabetes with vascular complications or more than 20 years duration **
- DVT or PE (unless anticoagulated) or current or personal history of ischemic heart disease**

- Multiple risk factors for arterial cardiovascular disease**
- Headaches with focal neurological symptoms ** or personal history of stroke
- Current or past history of breast cancer**
- Active viral hepatitis or mild or severe cirrhosis**
- Breast-feeding exclusively at the present time**
- Major surgery with immobilization within 1 month
- Personal history cholestasis with COC** or pregnancy

YES: history positive for one or more of above conditions

May not be able to use COCs

Consider non-estrogen methods: IUD, DMPA, POP, condoms, implant, diaphragm or cervical cap with spermicide, FAM, NFP, vasectomy or tubal sterilization

NO: history negative for all of above conditions

May use any sub-50-microgram COC* continuously or cyclically

Consider progestin only method POPs: (Micronor, Nor QD or Ovrette), Depo-Provera injections, implant or Mirena IUS, Copper T

Choose continuous or cyclic COC based on patient desires, availability, side effects, non-contraceptive benefits, cost, and prior experience of woman or clinician

- The World Health Organization and the Food and Drug Administration both recommend using the **lowest dose pill** that is effective. All combined pills with less than 50 µg of estrogen are effective and safe
- There are no studies demonstrating a decreased risk for deep vein thrombosis (DVT) in women on 20-µg pills. Data on higher dose pills have demonstrated that the less the estrogen dose, the lower the risk for DVT
- All COCs lower free testosterone. Class labeling in Canada for all combined pills states that use of pills may improve acne
- To minimize discontinuation due to spotting and breakthrough bleeding, warn women in advance, reassure that spotting and breakthrough bleeding become better over time. (See Figure 26.3, p. 107)

*The package insert for women on Yasmin states [Berlex-2001]: "Yasmin is different from other birth control pills because it contains the progestin drospirenone. Drospirenone may increase potassium. Therefore, you should not take Yasmin if you have kidney, liver or adrenal disease, because this could cause serious heart and health problems. Other drugs may also increase potassium. If you are currently on daily, long-term treatment for a chronic condition with any of the medications below, you should consult your healthcare provider about whether Yasmin is right for you, and during the first month that you take Yasmin, you should have a blood test to check your potassium level: NSAIDs (ibuprofen [Motrin®, Advil®], naproxen [Naprosyn®, Aleve®, and others] when taken long-term and daily for treatment of arthritis or other problems]; potassium-sparing diuretics (sprironolactone and others); potassium supplementation; ACE inhibitors (Capoten®, Vasotec®, Zestril® and others); Angiotensin-II receptor antagonists (Cozaar®, Diovan®, Avapro® and others); heparin"

**These are conditions that receive a WHO:3 or a WHO: 4 (See appendix pages A-5 and A-7)

Figure 26.3

SPOTTING/BREAKTHROUGH BLEEDING ON COCs 21/7*

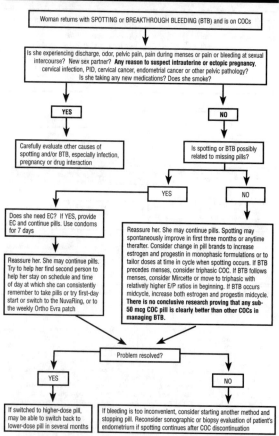

Woman returns with SPOTTING or BREAKTHROUGH BLEEDING (BTB) and is on COCs

Is she experiencing discharge, odor, pelvic pain, pain during menses or pain or bleeding at sexual intercourse? New sex partner? **Any reason to suspect intrauterine or ectopic pregnancy, cervical infection, PID, cervical cancer, endometrial cancer or other pelvic pathology? Is she taking any new medications? Does she smoke?**

YES

Carefully evaluate other causes of spotting and/or BTB, especially infection, pregnancy or drug interaction

NO

Is spotting or BTB possibly related to missing pills?

YES

Does she need EC? If YES, provide EC and continue pills. Use condoms for 7 days

Reassure her. She may continue pills. Try to help her find second person to help her stay on schedule and time of day at which she can consistently remember to take pills or try first-day start or switch to the NuvaRing, or to the weekly Ortho Evra patch

NO

Reassure her. She may continue pills. Spotting may spontaneously improve in first three months or anytime thereafter. Consider change in pill brands to increase estrogen and progestin in monophasic formulations or to tailor doses at time in cycle when spotting occurs. If BTB precedes menses, consider triphasic COC. If BTB follows menses, consider Mircette or move to triphasic with relatively higher E/P ratios in beginning. If BTB occurs midcycle, increase both estrogen and progestin midcycle. **There is no conclusive research proving that any sub-50 mcg COC pill is clearly better than other COCs in managing BTB.**

Problem resolved?

YES

If switched to higher-dose pill, may be able to switch back to lower-dose pill in several months

NO

If bleeding is too inconvenient, consider starting another method and stopping pill. Reconsider sonographic or biopsy evaluation of patient's endometrium if spotting continues after COC discontinuation

*See page 109 for comments on spotting/BTB in women on Seasonale (extended use of pills)

Figure 26.4

NEW ONSET OR WORSENING HEADACHES IN COC USERS

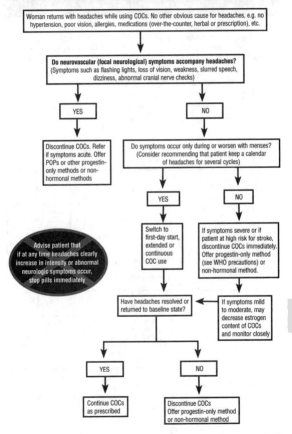

Woman returns with headaches while using COCs. No other obvious cause for headaches, e.g. no hypertension, poor vision, allergies, medications (over-the-counter, herbal or prescription), etc.

Do neurovascular (local neurological) symptoms accompany headaches?
(Symptoms such as flashing lights, loss of vision, weakness, slurred speech, dizziness, abnormal cranial nerve checks)

YES

Discontinue COCs. Refer if symptoms acute. Offer POPs or other progestin-only methods or non-hormonal methods.

NO

Do symptoms occur only during or worsen with menses?
(Consider recommending that patient keep a calendar of headaches for several cycles)

YES

Switch to first-day start, extended or continuous COC use

NO

If symptoms severe or if patient at high risk for stroke, discontinue COCs immediately. Offer progestin-only method (see WHO precautions) or non-hormonal method.

If symptoms mild to moderate, may decrease estrogen content of COCs and monitor closely

Advise patient that if at any time headaches clearly increase in intensity or abnormal neurologic symptoms occur, stop pills immediately

Have headaches resolved or returned to baseline state?

YES

Continue COCs as prescribed

NO

Discontinue COCs Offer progestin-only method or non-hormonal method

Figure 26.5

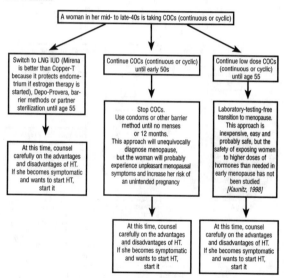

MAKING THE TRANSITION FROM COCs TO MENOPAUSE, WITH OR WITHOUT HORMONE THERAPY (HT)

The transition from COCs to menopause, with or without HT may be accomplished in a number of ways. Some reviewers of this algorithm switch to a 20 or 25-mcg pill if the patient is going to use COCs into the early 50s. Certainly a major concern must be unintended pregnancy. Work together to determine a method for pregnancy prevention that is acceptable and effective

This algorithm does NOT include testing for a woman's menopausal status using FSH or LH tests*

A woman in her mid- to late-40s is taking COCs (continuous or cyclic)

Switch to LNG IUD (Mirena is better than Copper-T because it protects endometrium if estrogen therapy is started), Depo-Provera, barrier methods or partner sterilization until age 55

Continue COCs (continuous or cyclic) until early 50s

Continue low dose COCs (continuous or cyclic) until age 55

At this time, counsel carefully on the advantages and disadvantages of HT. If she becomes symptomatic and wants to start HT, start it

Stop COCs. Use condoms or other barrier method until no menses or 12 months. This approach will unequivocally diagnose menopause, but the woman will probably experience unpleasant menopausal symptoms and increase her risk of an unintended pregnancy

Laboratory-testing-free transition to menopause. This approach is inexpensive, easy and probably safe, but the safety of exposing women to higher doses of hormones than needed in early menopause has not been studied [Kaunitz, 1998]

At this time, counsel carefully on the advantages and disadvantages of HT. If she becomes symptomatic and wants to start HT, start it

At this time, counsel carefully on the advantages and disadvantages of HT. If she becomes symptomatic and wants to start HT, start it

*FSH and LH testing are problematic because they show current status only. A perimenopausal woman can seem to be menopausal according to lab tests but ovulate unpredictably after that. See concerns about the provision of hormones to menopausal women on p. 23.

PATCHES - WEEKLY - ORTHO EVRA PATCH

DESCRIPTION: One Ortho Evra patch is worn for one week for each of 3 consecutive weeks, on the lower abdomen, buttocks, upper outer arm or to the upper torso (except for the breasts). The fourth week is patch-free to permit withdrawal bleeding. This 4.5 cm square patch delivers 20 micrograms of ethinyl estradiol and 150 mcg of the progestin, norelgestromin (the active metabolite of norgestimate) daily. *[Grimes-2001]* It takes 3 days to achieve steady states or plateau levels of hormones after application of the patch and the patch contains sufficent hormone for 9 days ◄

MECHANISM: The patch prevents pregnancy in the same manner as combined pills

COST: 3 patches are slightly more expensive than one cycle of brand pills

EFFECTIVENESS: Among perfect users (users who apply transdermal contraceptive patches on schedule and each patch remains in place for the full week), only 3-6 in 1,000 women (0.3-0.6%) are expected to become pregnant during the first year (Table 13.2 on p. 38). Pooled data from three contraceptive efficacy studies (22,155 treatment cycles) using life table analysis found an overall failure rate of about 1% (0.8% or 8 pregnancies per 1000 women through 13 cycles). *[Zieman-2001]*

In a multicenter trial of 1417 women randomized to use the patch (n=812) or the oral contraceptive, Triphasil (n=605), the pregnancy rate was lower (but not significantly lower) with the patch than with the pills. There were 5 pregnancies among women using the patch (1 user failure and 4 method failures). *[Audet-2001]* Of 15 pregnancies in the 3 clinical trials of the Ortho Evra Patch, 5 were in women who were markedly overweight (women more than 90 kilograms or 198 pounds). *[Zieman-2001]* (30% of failures in 3% of women) In an open-label study of 1,672 women receiving the Ortho Evra patch for 6 or 13 cycles, 6 pregnancies occurred, and 4 of them were in women weighing 90 kg or more *[Zieman-2001]*. There are no data available about typical failure rates. Correct and consistent use was significantly better among patch users compared to pill users. In randomized trials compliance was perfect in 88.2% of participants' cycles, significantly better than in women taking pills (in 77.7% of women's cycles on pills compliance was perfect). *[Audet 2001]*

ADVANTAGES

Menstrual: Like combined pills

Sexual/Psychological:
- May enhance sexual enjoyment due to diminished fear of pregnancy
- Attractive for women who forget to take pills
- Does not interrupt intercourse

Cancers/tumors and masses: No data yet; benefits probably quite comparable to combined pills

Other:
- Option throughout the reproductive years: Age is not a reason to avoid the Patch. Compliance among teens using patch is good. For some women compliance may be easier than taking a pill every day *[Audet-2001]*. Each patch contains enough hormone to suppress ovulation for up to 9 days.
- May bathe, swim and do normal activities

DISADVANTAGES

Menstrual: In the first cycle about one-fifth of patch users experienced breakthrough bleeding or spotting. There were no statistically significant differences between the patch and COCs with regard to breakthrough bleeding in any cycle in the randomized trial of the patch vs Triphasil. *[Audet 2001]*

Sexual/Psychological: Similar to pills, but use may be more obvious than pills. See p. 102
Cancers/tumors and masses: Same as COCs
Other:

- Lack of protection against sexually transmitted infections (STIs)
- Among 812 women on the patch, 3 serious adverse events were considered possible or likely related to use of the patch, including 1 case of pain and paraesthesia in the left arm, 1 case of migraine and 1 case of cholecystitis *[Audet-2001]*
- Must remove and replace patch weekly. Application site problems include partial detachment (2.8%) or complete detachment (1.8%) and skin irritation (1.1%) *[Audet-2001]*. **Hyperpigmentation has been noted under the site of patch application.** In a study of patch wear under conditions of physical exertion and variable temperatures and humidity, less than 2% of patches were replaced for complete or partial detachment. 2.6% of women discontinued using the patch because of application site reactions. Problems did not increase over time *[Audet-2001]*. Border of patch may become dirty, picking up lint, hairs or fabric. Able to remove with baby oil after patch is changed
- Nausea occurred in 20.4% of women on patch vs 18.3% of women using oral contraceptives; patch was discontinued by 1.8% of women because of nausea *[Audet-2001]*
- Breast discomfort was greater in women using the patch than in women on the pill. The difference was significant only in cycles 1 and 2 (15.4% vs 3.5% in cycle 1 and 6.6% vs 1.5% in cycle 2). For cycles 3-13, breast discomfort occurred in 0 to 3.2% of women using the patch and in 0 to 1.7% of women on pills (not statistically significant) *[Audet-2001]*
- Headaches were as likely in women on patch (21.9%) as in women on pills (22.1%)
- Irritation or an allergic skin reaction while using the patch (19%) ◀

COMPLICATIONS (See p. 104)

PRESCRIBING PRECAUTIONS

- Precautions for the patch are the same as those for combined pills (see page 106)
- **Women weighing more than 90 kg (198 lbs)** should be told that the patch may be less effective and that they should consider using a backup. Should not be a "first-line" ◀ method for woman over 198 pounds without backup

CANDIDATES FOR USE

- Women wanting to avoid daily pill-taking or a sex-related method like condoms
- Women wanting regular menstrual periods. May be used by individuals allergic to latex

Adolescents: **Excellent option, particularly for teenage women unable to remember to take pills daily** *[Archer-2002]*

INITIATING METHOD:

- With the 1st pack of patches, the patient is eligible for up to three free replacement patches. Write prescription for "replacement patch" with the first box of patches
- **A pelvic examination is not necessary prior to starting this method** *[Stewart-2001]*
- Ask patient, "What day of the week is the easiest for you to remember?" and start then if you are reasonably certain she is not pregnant
- It is usually recommended that the first patch be placed on the first day of the next menstrual period. If started any other day, use a backup contraceptive for 7 days
- Women switching from pills can switch to the patch any time in cycle. They need not wait to complete pack of pills
- Women switching from DMPA should start when the next injection is due
- But as with pills, the patch can be started anytime with backup for 7 days, if you are reasonably sure the woman is not pregnant

INSTRUCTIONS FOR PATIENT
- If the PATCH-FREE interval is more than 9 days (late restart), apply a new patch and use backup contraception for 7 days
- No band-aids, tatoos, or decals on top of patch as this might alter absorption of hormones
- Smooth the edges down when you first put it on
- Avoid placing patch on exactly the same site 2 consecutive weeks
- Location of patch should not be altered in mid-week
- Women should check the patch daily to make sure all edges remain closely adherent to skin
- Single replacement patches are available through pharmacists. The manufacturer will reimburse a woman for up to $12 for the replacement patch
- Disposal: fold over self. Place in solid waste, preferably in a sealed plastic bag to minimize hormone leakage into waste site. Do not flush down toilet

FOLLOW UP
- What is happening to your menstrual periods?
- Have you experienced skin irritation?
- Has your patch ever come off partially or completely?
- Have you had problems remembering to replace your patch on schedule

COMPLICATIONS (See p. 104)
- An allergic reaction while using the patch

PROBLEM MANAGEMENT (See p. 113)
FERTILITY AFTER DISCONTINUATION OF METHOD: Likely the same excellent return of fertility as COCs

INJECTIONS – MONTHLY – LUNELLE

Although NOT currently available in the USA, Lunelle is a 0.5 cc suspension containing 25 mg medroxyprogesterone acetate and 5 mg estradiol cypionate injected intramuscularly into the deltoid or gluteus maximus muscle every 28 ± 5 days (ideally every 28-30 days). Brand names: Lunelle, Lunella, Cylco-Provera, Cyclofem, Ciclofemina, Feminena and HRP 112.

VAGINAL CONTRACEPTIVE RING - MONTHLY - NuvaRing

DESCRIPTION: (also see www.nuvaring.com) The NuvaRing is a combined hormonal contraceptive consisting of a 5.4 cm (2 inches) diameter flexible (not hard) ring, 4 mm (1/8 inch) in thickness. The ring is made of ethylene vinylacetate polymer. It is left in place in the vagina for 3 weeks (or 1 month) and then removed for a week to allow withdrawal bleeding. It may be used continuously with no hormone-free days, but this is not approved (off-label). **It is generally recommended that it not be removed for intercourse. If it must be, however, it should be replaced within 3 hours.** Douching is discouraged but topical therapies (antifungal agents, spermicides, etc) are allowed. NuvaRing releases low doses of ethinyl estradiol (15 micrograms daily) and etonogestrel, the active form of desogestrel (120 micrograms daily). With oral hormones there is a daily spike in hormone levels after the woman swallows each dose, followed by a gradual drop throughout the rest of the day. A single vaginal ring maintains a steady, low release rate for 35 days while in place and releases less estrogen daily at a steadier rate than pills or patches

MECHANISM: *contraceptive effects similar to combined pills*. This method suppresses ovulation for 35 days, therefore method is forgiving if a woman is forgetful [Mulders-2001]. Also see COCs, p. 97

COST: Each ring costs approximately the same as one cycle of pills. It is possible to get some free rings via the website at www.nuvaring.com. Large programs pay as little as $3 for each ◄ NuvaRing.

EFFECTIVENESS: Overall pregnancy rate of 0.3 [Trussell-2004] to 0.65 [Roumen-2001] per 100 woman-years (all first-year users). There is no information about typical use failure rate, so a typical use failure rate of 8% is used by Trussell in the 18th edition of *Contraceptive Technology* (same figure as for combined pills). It is likely that since the method needs to ◄ be remembered once per month rather than once per day, that the typical user failure rate would be lower

ADVANTAGES: No daily fluctuation in hormone levels ◄
Menstrual:
- Withdrawal bleeding occurs in 98.5% of cycles, and bleeding at other times in only 5.5% of cycles [Dieben-2002]; much better withdrawal/spotting pattern than COCs probably due to NOT forgetting pills and the steady even blood levels that are achieved
- Irregular bleeding is low in the first cycle of use (6%) and continues to be low throughout subsequent cycles [Dieben-2002]

Sexual/Psychological: Decreased fear of pregnancy may increase pleasure from intercourse
Cancers/tumors and masses: No published data; probably similar to COCs
Other: There are only 2 tasks for ring users to remember: insertion and removal once a month so compliance may be easier (92% vs. 75% for pills in one study) [Bjarnadottir-2002]
- 85% of women and 71% of partners say they cannot feel it [Dieben-2002]
- The lowest serum levels of estrogen and progestin in any combined hormonal method
- Privacy - no visible patch or pill packages. Particularly helpful for some teens ◄

DISADVANTAGES
Menstrual: Withdrawal bleeding continued beyond the ring-free interval in about one quarter of cycles (20% to 27%) [Roumen-2001]. However, most of the time it is just spotting. Although not necessary, some women may rinse the ring. Also, ring can be accidentally ◄ pulled out by a tampon
Sexual/Psychological: Some women dislike placing/removing objects into/out of vagina Some women or men may feel ring during intercourse. If bothersome, ring may be ◄ removed and reinserted within 3 hours
Cancers/tumors and masses: None
Other: Adverse events reported by vaginal contraceptive ring users that were judged by the investigators to be device related are headache (6.6%), nausea (2.8%), weight increase (2.2%), dysmenorrhea (1.8%), depression (1.7%), leukorrhea (5.3%), vaginitis (5.0%), and vaginal discomfort (2.2%) [Roumen-2001]

COMPLICATIONS: Similar to combined pills

PRESCRIBING PRECAUTIONS
- The WHO Medical Eligibility Criteria for the NuvaRing are the same as for combined pills
- Women who are hesitant about touching their genitalia or who have difficulty inserting or removing ring may not be good candidates
- Women with pronounced pelvic relaxation

CANDIDATES

- Women wanting to avoid having to do something daily, or at the time of intercourse
- Women wanting regular menstrual periods

Adolescents: Excellent option; requires less discipline than taking pills daily

INITIATING METHOD: *Best approach - teach women to insert and remove ring in office.* *Ask women if they would like you to insert a ring after you do a Pap smear to* *demonstrate just how little she will feel the ring* ⬅

- A new ring is inserted any time during the first 5 days of a normal menstrual cycle and backup for 7 days is recommended in package insert
- New ring can be inserted at any time in cycle if reasonably certain woman is not pregnant; use backup x 7 days (off-label)

INSTRUCTIONS FOR PATIENT

- The package insert states that backup must be used during the first 7 days that the first ring is in place
- The NuvaRing is removed at the end of 3 weeks of wear; then, after one ring-free week, the woman inserts a new ring
- The woman's menstrual period (withdrawal bleed) occurs during the ring-free week
- Ring removal during intercourse is not recommended; however, women who want to remove it during intercourse may do so without having to use a backup method as long as it is not removed for longer than 3 hours a day
- No special accuracy is required for ring placement; absorption is fine from anywhere in the vagina
- Because the ring is small and flexible, **most women do not notice any pressure or discomfort**, and it is not likely to be uncomfortable for their partners during intercourse
- Always have 2 rings on hand in case one is lost
- Avoid douching with ring in place ⬅
- Rings may be stored at room temperature avoiding extreme heat for up to 4 months. ⬅ If a woman has more than a 4-month supply of rings, they may be stored in a refrigerator. Rings kept in a refrigerator should not freeze
- A ring that falls into the toilet does float! It can be washed with soap and water and reinserted ⬅
- If the ring is left in place longer than three weeks, the user is probably still protected from pregnancy for up to 35 days by the same ring, allowing clinicians flexibility in how often ⬅ they tell women the ring must be replaced. For example, the ring could be reinserted on the first of the month each month with no hormone-free interval (similar to taking combined pills with no hormone-free days). (Obviously off-label, but extended cycle use is under study) Or rings could be removed and a new one reinserted each month on the date of the month the woman was born
- **Dispose of ring with solid waste, preferably in a sealed plastic bag to minimize** ⬅ **leakage into waste site**

FOLLOW UP: Ask about difficulty during removal or insertion. Women may need closer follow-up if they have: genital prolapse, severe constipation, or frequent vaginal infection (i.e. recurrent yeast infection). Otherwise, similar to women on pills

FERTILITY AFTER DISCONTINUATION: Presumably excellent and immediate

CHAPTER 27

Progestin-Only Contraceptives
www.managingcontraception.com

The progestin-only methods are progestin-only pills (p. 124), Depo-Provera (p. 128), Implanon (p. 137), and Jadelle (p. 139). The LNG IUD is described on p. 91

LOW DOSE PROGESTIN PILLS – DAILY – often called MINI-PILLS OR POPS

DESCRIPTION: Progestin-only pills (POPs) are also known as mini-pills. POPs contain only a progestin and are taken daily with no hormone-free days. POPs have lower progestin doses than combined pills and no estrogen. Each tablet of Micronor and Nor-QD contains 0.35 mg norethindrone. Each tablet of Ovrette has 0.075 mg of norgestrel.

EFFECTIVENESS *[Trussell J IN Contraceptive Technology 2004]*
Perfect use failure rate in first year: 0.3% (See Table 13.2, p. 39)
(if 300 women take POPs for 1 year, only 1 will become pregnant in the first year of perfect use)
Typical use failure rate in first year: 8.0%

MECHANISM: Thickens cervical mucus to prevent sperm entry into upper reproductive tract (major mechanism). Effect short lived - requires punctual dosing. Other mechanisms include ovulation suppression (in about 50% of cycles), thin, atrophic endometrium which inhibits implantation; and slowed diminished mobility. Some POPs in Europe suppress ◀— ovulation more than the levonorgestrel, norgestrel and norethindrone pills used in the USA

COST *[Trussell, 1995; Smith, 1993]*
• POPs cost more than combined pills both in pharmacies and in sales to public programs

ADVANTAGES
Menstrual:
  • Decreased menstrual blood loss, cramps and pain, amenorrhea (10% of women).
    Amenorrhea is more likely with punctual dosing
  • Decrease in ovulatory pain (Mittelschmerz) in cycles when ovulation suppressed
Sexual/physiological:
  • May enhance sexual enjoyment due to diminished fear of pregnancy
  • No disruption at time of intercourse; facilitates spontaneity
Cancers, tumors and masses:
  • Possible protection against endometrial cancer
Other:
  • Rapid return to baseline fertility
  • Possible reduction in PID risk due to cervical mucus thickening
  • Good option for women who cannot use estrogen but want to take pills
  • May be used by smokers over age 35. **Discourage smoking, of course!**
  • May be used by breastfeeding women

DISADVANTAGES

Menstrual: Irregular menses ranging from amenorrhea to increased days of spotting and bleeding but with reduced blood loss overall

Sexual/psychological:
- Spotting and bleeding may interfere with sexual activity
- Intermittent amenorrhea may raise concerns about pregnancy
- Possible increase in depression, anxiety, irritability, fatigue or other mood changes, but often POPs reduce risk of these disorders

Cancers, tumors and masses:
- May be associated with slightly higher risk of persistent ovarian follicles

Other:
- Must take pill at same time each day (more than 3-hour delay considered by some clinicians to be equivalent to a "missed pill")
- Effect on cervical mucus decreases after 22 hours and is gone after 27 hours
- No protection against STIs

COMPLICATIONS

- Allergy to progestin pill is rare
- Amenorrheic, Latina, breast-feeding women who had gestational diabetes may be at higher risk of developing overt diabetes in first year postpartum *[Kjos, 1998]*

CANDIDATES FOR USE (See 2004 WHO Medical Eligibility Criteria, A-1 - A-8)

- Virtually every woman who can take pills on a daily basis can be a candidate for POPs
- POPs are particularly good for women with contraindications to or side effects from estrogen:
  - Women with personal history of thrombosis
  - Recently postpartum women
  - Women who are exclusively breast-feeding
  - Smokers over age 35
  - Women who had or fear chloasma, worsening migraine headaches, hypertriglyceridemia or other estrogen-related side effects
  - Women with hypertension, coronary artery disease or cerebrovascular disease
  - Women wth lupus ←

PRESCRIBING PRECAUTIONS

Progestin-only pills can be used by all women willing and able to take daily pills except:
- Suspected or demonstrated pregnancy (although there are no proven harmful effects for the fetus)
- Current breast cancer or breast cancer less than 5 years ago (WHO:3)
- Active hepatitis, hepatic failure, jaundice
- Inability to absorb sex steroids from gastrointestinal tract (active colitis, etc.)
- Taking medications that increase hepatic clearance (rifampin, and the anticonvulsants carbamazepine, oxcarbazepine, phenytoin (Dilantin), phenobarbital, primidone, topiramate and felbamate, (not valproic acid), St. Johns Wort or griseofulvin). Efficacy ← in combination with Orlistat and other fat-binding agents is not well studied

MEDICAL ELIGIBILITY CHECKLIST: Evidence-based criteria for deciding whether women with 130 different conditions are presented in the appendix, pages A-1 through A-8. These criteria were updated at the World Health Organization in 2004. Ask the client the questions below. If she answers YES to a question below, follow the instructions; in some cases she can still use POPs

1. Do you think you are pregnant?

☐ No ☐ Yes   Assess if pregnant. If she might be pregnant, give her latex male condoms to use until reasonably sure that she is not pregnant. Then she can start POPs

2. Do you have or have you ever had breast cancer? (See page A4)

☐ No ☐ Yes   Do not provide POPs. Help her choose a method without hormones. May possibly consider POPs or DMPA if disease-free x 5 years (WHO:3)

3. Do you have jaundice, severe cirrhosis of the liver, acute liver infection or tumor? (Are your eyes or skin unusually yellow?) (See page A7)

☐ No ☐ Yes   Perform physical exam and arrange lab tests or refer. If she has serious active liver disease (jaundice, painful or enlarged liver, viral hepatitis, liver tumor), may ◄ be able to use POPs with more intensive follow-up (WHO:3)

4. Do you have vaginal bleeding that is unusual for you? (See page A4)

☐ No ☐ Yes   If she is not pregnant but has unexplained vaginal bleeding that suggests an underlying medical condition, can provide POPs since neither the underlying condition nor its assessment will be affected. Promptly assess and treat any underlying condition as appropriate, or refer. Reassess POP use based on findings

5. Are you taking medicine for seizures? Taking rifampin (rifampicin), griseofulvin or aminoglutethimide? St. Johns Wort? (See page A8)

☐ No ☐ Yes   If she is taking phenytoin, carbamazepine, barbiturate, topiramate, oxycarbamazepine, or primidone for seizures or rifampin, griseofulvin, aminoglutethamide or St. John's Wort, provide condoms or spermicide or help her choose another method that is more effective, such as DMPA. Use of valproic acid does NOT lower the effectiveness of POPs. Discuss ECPs

6. Do you have problems with severe diarrhea from Crohn's disease or other bowel disorders? Or are you using medications that block fat absorption?

☐ No ☐ Yes   Help her choose a non-oral method of birth control

SPECIAL SITUATIONS

History of pregnancy while using POPs correctly:

- Consider DMPA or switch to IUD or to estrogen containing method
- Continue POPs but add condoms or other backup with every act of coitus

Use with a broad-spectrum antibiotic such as tetracycline or erythromycin:

- Few studies support antibiotic's role in contraceptive failure. See 2004 WHO Medical Eligibility Criteria for "other antibiotics", WHO:1, Page A8. Some clinicians encourage backup for first 1-2 weeks, others for full duration of antibiotic use. Explain conflicting advice now being given; let patient decide whether to use backup method.

INITIATING METHOD

- **A pelvic examination is not necessary prior to initiation of this method** *[Stewart-2001]*
- *New starts:* Offer condoms either for back-up for 7 days or for use should patient stop POPs. Also offer advance prescription of PLAN B or give her a package of PLAN B
- *Post-partum:* May initiate immediately regardless of breast-feeding status (PPFA, UCSF, Grady Memorial Hospital)
  Note: WHO and IPPF are concerned about theoretical impact of POPs on breast milk production and recommend waiting until 6 weeks to initiate use of DMPA and POPs
- *After miscarriage or abortion:* Start immediately
- *Menstruating women:* Start on menses if possible. May initiate anytime in cycle if woman is not pregnant, but recommend at least 1-week back-up barrier method
- *Switching from IUD, COCs, DMPA, to POPs:* start immediately. Need for back-up depends on previous method used: **IUD:** start immediately, backup for 7 days; Some clinicians say 48 hours minimum; others say no backup. **COCs:** start immediately if cycle of hormonally active pills completed; backup not necessary if no pill-free interval. **DMPA:** start immediately if switching at or before next DMPA injection due (no backup necessary)

INSTRUCTIONS FOR PATIENT

- Take one pill daily at same time each day until end of pack. Start next pack the next day
- If at risk for infection, use condoms with every act of intercourse
- If you miss a pill by more than 3 hours from regular time, take the missed pill(s) and use backup for 48 hours. Consider using emergency contraception if sex in past 3-5 days. Obtain a package of Plan B to have at home in case of a mistake ◄—

FOLLOW-UP

- How many pills do you typically miss or are late taking per week? Per pack?
- Have you missed any pills in last 3 days? (candidate for EC)
- Have you missed any periods or experienced any symptoms of pregnancy?
- What has your menstrual bleeding been like?
- Have you had any increase in headaches, or change in mood or libido?
- Do you plan to have children? OR Do you plan to have more children?
- What are you doing to protect yourself from STIs?

PROBLEM MANAGEMENT

- *Amenorrhea:* Rule out pregnancy with first episode or whenever symptoms of pregnancy noted. Otherwise, amenorrhea is not harmful when women take progestin-only pills
- *Irregular bleeding:* After finding out if missing pills, rule out STIs, pregnancy, cancer. If not at risk and no evidence of underlying pathology, reassure patient; 3-day course of high dose NSAIDS may help
- *Heavy bleeding:* Rule out STIs, pregnancy, cancer. If no evidence of underlying pathology, rule out clinically significant anemia. Trial of 3 days high dose NSAIDS. If fails, may need estrogen-containing contraceptives (addition of physiologic doses ET only may compromise cervical mucus barrier), Mirena IUS or non-hormonal methods of contraception ◄—
- *Abdominal pain:* Consider pelvic pathology (ectopic pregnancy, torsion, appendicitis, PID) and refer for treatment. If ovarian cyst is cause, it may usually be managed conservatively unless pain is severe. Progestin slows follicular atresia. Recheck in 6 weeks and anytime her symptoms worsen

FERTILITY AFTER DISCONTINUATION OF METHOD: Fertility returns to its
baseline levels promptly

DMPA INJECTIONS (DEPO-PROVERA) - EACH 3 MONTHS

DESCRIPTION: 1 cc of a crystalline suspension of 150 mg depot medroxyprogesterone acetate injected intramuscularly into the deltoid or gluteus maximus muscle every 11-13 weeks For more information, call 1-800-253-8600 ext. 38244. Depo-Provera Subcutaneous - 104, subcutaneous injections of 104 mg of DMPA facilitate women giving themselves Depo-Provera injections at home. Women receive up to 14 weeks of contraceptive protection from an injection of 104 mg of DMPA SQ ◄◄

EFFECTIVENESS *[Trussell J IN Contraceptive Technology - 2004]*
• Approved labeling indicates each injection effective for up to 13 weeks
Perfect use failure rate in first year: 0.3% (See Table 13.2, p. 39)
Typical use failure rate in first year: 3%
Continuation at 1 year: 23% *[Westfall-1996]* 42% *[Polaneczky-1996]* 56% *[Trussell-2004]* ◄

Subcutaneous Depo-Provera ◄

Despite the lower dose of Sub Q DMPA (104 vs 150 mg), no pregnancies occurred among the 44% of study subjects who were overweight (26%) or obese (18%). In fact, there were no pregnancies at all in 720 women over one year. 55% were amenorrheic at the end of one year. *[Jain J, Jakimiuk AJ et all-2004]*

MECHANISMS: Suppresses ovulation by inhibiting LH and FSH surge, thickens cervical mucus blocking sperm entry into female upper reproductive tract, slows tubal and endometrial mobility, and causes thinning of the endometrium

COST: In Washington State, health departments pay $4.75 for 28 days of contraception for a woman receiving Depo-Provera each 3 months. This is 4 times greater than the cost of pills for the same clinics, $1.35 per cycle. *[Margulies - 2001]* The co-pay for DMPA is about $60/vial

ADVANTAGES
Menstrual:
• Less menstrual blood loss, anemia, or hemorrhagic corpus luteum cysts
• After 1 year of use, 50% of women develop amenorrhea; 80% develop amenorrhea in 5 years. For this to be an advantage, it must be clearly explained at first and subsequent visits. See discussion of structured counseling on page 14
• Decreased menstrual cramps, pain and ovulation pain
• Improvement in endometriosis. *Depo-Provera Subcutaneous 104* received formal ◄ FDA approval for management of endometriosis pain on March 29, 2005
Sexual/psychological:
• Intercourse may be more pleasurable without worry of pregnancy
• Convenient; permits spontaneous sexual activity; requires no action at time of intercourse
Cancers, tumors, and masses:
• Significant reduction in risk of endometrial cancer
• Possible reduction in risk of ovarian cancer
Benefits for women with medical problems:
• Suppresses ovulation, bleeding and menstrual blood loss in anticoagulated women and women with bleeding diathesis; decreases anemia
• Reduces acute sickle cell crises by 70% *[de Abood-1997]*
• Excellent method for women on anticonvulsant drugs; may actually decrease seizures and effectiveness not compromised
• Amenorrhea and prolonged effective contraception may be very important for severely developmentally or physically challenged women. One reviewer makes home visits for some wheelchair bound patients who love Depo-Provera

128

Other:
- The drop in teen pregnancies in 1990s, abortions and births, is attributed to Depo-Provera, Norplant, EC, condoms and abstinence promoting programs
- Significantly reduces risk for ectopic pregnancies and slightly decrease risk of PID
- Convenient: single injection provides at least 13 weeks protection
- Most protocols call for administration anytime between 11 and 13 weeks. However, DMPA is usually forgiving of late injections
- Less user-dependent than POPs, COCs
- Good option for women who cannot use estrogen (see CANDIDATES FOR USE)
- Private: no visible clue that patient is using except for impact on menses
- May be used by nursing mothers
- Return to baseline fertility may be delayed, but is excellent ←

DISADVANTAGES
Menstrual:
- Irregular menses during first several months: many women experience unpredictable spotting and bleeding, occasionally blood loss reported to be heavy but unlikely to cause anemia. After 6-12 months, amenorrhea more likely (50% after 1 year)

Sexual/psychological: Also see weight gain, below
- Spotting and bleeding may interfere with sexual activity
- Amenorrhea may raise patient's fears of pregnancy or build-up of menses in uterus if not explained well
- Hypoestrogenism can (infrequently) cause dyspareunia, hot flashes or decreased libido
- Possible increase in depression, anxiety, irritation, PMS, fatigue or other mood changes, but often DMPA reduces risk of these disorders
- Fear of needles may make this an unacceptable choice

Cancers, tumors, and masses: none
Other: (See boxed message: Depo Provera & Bones on p. 130)
- No protection against STIs: must use condoms if at risk
- Must return every 11-13 weeks for injection (difficult for some women) or get injection from person trained to provide injections ←
- Long acting: *not* immediately reversible
- Slow to return to baseline fertility: average 10 months from last injection
- Occasionally, hypoestrogenism ($E_2 < 25$) may develop as a result of FSH suppression. Potential for decreased bone mineral density if used for prolonged period without opportunity for recovery prior to menopause. May have more effect on teen bones
- Severe headaches may occur - rarely attributable to DMPA
- Acne, hirsutism may develop
- Possible increase in diabetes risk in amenorrheic breastfeeding women with diagnosis of gestational diabetes during first year postpartum *[Kjos 1999]*
- Metabolic impacts: glucose (slight rise), LDL (slight rise or neutral), HDL (may decrease)
- Other hormone-related Sx: breast tenderness, bloating, hair loss, vasomotor symptoms

COMPLICATIONS
- Progressive significant weight gain possible. Average of 5.4 lbs in first year and 16.5 lbs at 5 yrs *[Schwallie-1973]* See p. 132: WEIGHT GAIN: A TEACHABLE MOMENT. Weight gain is more of a problem for teenagers who are already obese when they start receiving Depo-Provera injections
- Severe depression (rare) (average MMPI does not change in women on DMPA).
- Severe allergic reaction, including anaphylaxis (very rare). May consider having women wait in or near office for 20 minutes after injection. (Reviewers disagree about this recommendation, especially for previous DMPA users). Ask patients to report itching at injection site

CANDIDATES FOR USE (See new (2004) WHO Criteria on pages A-1 through A-8)
- Women who want intermediate-to-long-term contraception and can return every 11-13 weeks
- Women who do not plan a pregnancy soon after DMPA discontinuation
- Women who want privacy, convenience, and high efficacy
- Women who want or need to avoid estrogen:
  - Women with personal history of thrombosis (WHO: 2) or strong family history of venous thromboembolism (WHO: 1)
  - Recently postpartum women (WHO: 1)
  - Women who are exclusively breast-feeding beyond 6 weeks postpartum (WHO: 1). There is debate about use of DMPA in breastfeeding women less than 6 weeks PP (see p. 132 under INITIATING METHOD POSTPARTUM)
  - Smokers over age 35 (WHO: 1)
  - Women who fear chloasma or had vomiting, migraine headaches, hypertriglyceridemia, or other estrogen-related side effects
  - Women who use drugs which affect liver clearance (except aminoglutethimide)
  - Women with anemia, fibroids, seizure disorder (WHO 1), sickle cell disease (WHO: 1), endometriosis, hypertriglyceridemia (WHO: 2), systemic lupus erythematosus or coagulation disorder (hyper- or hypo-coagulation)
  - Physically compromised women for whom bleeding is a nuisance or a problem

Adolescent women: (WHO: 2) Only 4 things to do each year! ←
- Extremely effective with long carry-over if patient returns late for reinjection (see Figure 27.1, p. 135); Decreases menstrual cramps and pain
- Privacy and confidentiality possible
- For some teens may be only acceptable method
- May be associated with significant weight gain, acne, complexion changes
- Requires periodic reinjections

Bone Mineral Density and Depo-Provera

Women who used DMPA for more than 2 years have significantly reduced bone mineral density (BMD) of lumbar spine and femoral neck. But effect is largely reversible, even after ≥ 4 years of DMPA use, comparable to the effect and reversal seen after lactation *[Petitti-2000]*. **All women using DMPA including teens should be taking in sufficient calcium in diet or be encouraged to take calcium supplements. Also encourage to exercise regularly and avoid smoking.** A double-blind randomized controlled study of estrogen supplementation in ← adolescent girls demonstrated at 24 months of DMPA use an increase of 4.7% in femoral neck bone density in teenagers receiving monthly injecions of estradiol cypronate (5 mg) and a decrease of 5.1% in femoral neck bone density in teens provided DMPA and monthly placebo injections of 5 ml normal saline *[Cromer-2005]*. Bone mass may return after Depo-Provera has been discontinued. Cromer et al indicate that they "cannot conclude that observed bone loss is irreversible until further study is conducted and the relevant data have been obtained." *[Cromer-2005]* Subcutaneous DMPA did NOT decrease bone density ←

PRESCRIBING PRECAUTIONS: Women unwilling to accept a change in their menstrual periods
- Pregnancy
- Undiagnosed abnormal vaginal bleeding
- Unable to tolerate injections; afraid of shots
- History of breast cancer, MI or stroke

- Blood pressure >160 systolic or > 100 diastolic
- Current venous thromboembolism (unless anticoagulated)
- Active viral hepatitis
- Known hypersensitivity to Depo-Provera
New package insert black box warning

DRUG INTERACTIONS: Aminoglutethimide (Cytodren), used to treat Cushings disease, reduces DMPA efficacy

MEDICAL ELIGIBILITY CHECKLIST
Ask the client the questions below. If she answers NO to ALL the questions, then she CAN use DMPA if she wants. If she answers YES to a question below, follow the instructions

1. Do you think you are pregnant?

☐ No ☐ Yes   Assess if pregnant. If she might be pregnant, give her condoms or spermicide to use until reasonably sure that she is not pregnant. Then she can start DMPA

2. Do you plan to become pregnant in the next year?

☐ No ☐ Yes   Use another method with less potential delay in return of fertility

3. Do you have serious medical problems such as heart attack, severe chest pain, or uncontrolled high blood pressure? Have you ever had such problems? (See pages A-3 and A-4)

☐ No ☐ Yes   In general, do not provide DMPA if she reports heart attack (WHO:3), stroke (WHO:3), heart disease due to blocked arteries, severe high blood pressure (systolic ≥ 160 or diastolic ≥ 100)(WHO:3), diabetes for more than 20 years (WHO:3), or damage to vision, kidneys, or nervous system caused by diabetes or by HTN. Help her choose another effective method. All the above conditions receive a "3" in the 2001 WHO Medical Eligibility Criteria

4. Do you have or have you recently had breast cancer (WHO: 3 or 4)? (See page A-5)

☐ No ☐ Yes   Do not provide DMPA. Help her choose a method without hormones. If cancer-free for 5 or more years, a woman with a history of breast cancer may possibly use DMPA (WHO: 3)

5. Do you have jaundice, cirrhosis of the liver, a liver infection or tumor? (Are her eyes or skin unusually yellow?) (See page A-7)

☐ No ☐ Yes   Perform physical exam or refer. If she has serious liver disease (jaundice, painful or enlarged liver, viral hepatitis, liver tumor), do not provide DMPA. Refer for care. Help her choose a method without hormones

6. Do you have vaginal bleeding that is unusual for you? (See page A-4)

☐ No ☐ Yes   If she is not pregnant but has unexplained vaginal bleeding that suggest a serious underlying medical condition (WHO:3), assess and treat any underlying condition as appropriate, or refer. Provide DMPA based on findings

INITIATING METHOD (see Figure 27.1, page 135)

A pelvic exam is NOT necessary prior to the initiation of this method *[Stewart-2001]*

Cycling women:
- Preferred start time is during first 5 days from the start of menses
- Alternative: inject anytime in the cycle if not pregnant, back-up x 7 days (see 27.1)

Postpartum women: May give injection prior to hospital discharge. Special considerations:
- After severe obstetrical blood loss, delay injection until lochia stops
- If woman has history or high risk for severe postpartum depression, observe carefully and delay injection at least 4-6 weeks
- Breast-feeding women: May either start DMPA immediately or wait 4-6 week.

Women who have spontaneous or therapeutic abortion: May initiate immediately.

Women switching methods:
- May start anytime patient is known not to be pregnant
- Hormonal method: if she has been using her current method consistently and ◄──── correctly, may initiate immediately
- If switching from non-hormonal method, offer same options as cycling women

INSTRUCTIONS FOR PATIENT: *Some women may be able to give themselves Depo-Provera injections*

- Do NOT massage area where shot was given for a few hours (massaging area may reduce duration of action and thereby effectiveness)
- Expect irregular bleeding/spotting in beginning. Usually decreases over time. Return at any time spotting or bleeding is bothersome. Rx may make bleeding pattern more tolerable
- It is not harmful or dangerous if you do not have periods while you use DMPA

WEIGHT GAIN: A TEACHABLE MOMENT

When you see a patient who is very heavy or has gained enough weight to disturb her, you have a teachable moment. BE PREPARED FOR THAT TEACHABLE MOMENT.

Help someone to lose weight in 60 seconds! Encourage her to program her life to:

1. **Eat less** (small, frequent meals helps some to lose weight); eat balanced diet with lots of fruits and vegetables and minimal fats, chips, cookies, pasta and other carbohydrates
2. **Exercise more**...and every day
3. Find patterns of eating and exercising that you enjoy! You won't do them for long unless you enjoy the process.
4. Call Overeaters Anonymous (OA), a free source of love and caring. OA works! www.overeatersanonymous.org
5. Drink 8-10 glasses of water daily

- Be sure to take in 1000 mg (women over age 25) to 1200 mg (adolescent women) of calcium every day to build your bones. Take calcium tablets like calcium carbonate or TUMS daily if your diet does not include enough calcium. Calcium is best absorbed when 500 mg is taken late in the day with a glass of orange juice. Get weight bearing and muscle-strengthening exercise at least 3 times a week (preferably 20 minutes daily)
- Return in 11-13 weeks for your next injection. Use abstinence, condoms, and EC, if necessary, if you are late coming for your re-injection (more than 13 weeks)
- Pregnancy is rare; return if you develop pregnancy symptoms other than amenorrhea
- Serious complications with DMPA are rare, but return if you develop severe headaches; heavy bleeding; depression or problems at the shot site (pus, pain, allergic reaction)

FOLLOW-UP

- Are you experiencing spotting or irregular bleeding? Have you missed periods or had very light periods? Are you concerned about your pattern of bleeding?
- Did you have pain at the injection site after previous injection?
- Have you felt depressed or had major mood changes?
- Have you gained 5 pounds or more? (See WEIGHT GAIN, A TEACHABLE MOMENT, p. 132) Be sure to weigh patients at each visit. This means at **each and every visit**
- Do you have any increase in your headaches?
- Have you had the feeling that you may be pregnant?
- Did you have any problems returning on time for this injection?
- Do you plan to have children? OR Do you plan to have more children?
- **What are you doing to protect yourself from STIs? When appropriate encourage condom use**

STRUCTURED COUNSELING FOR DEPO-PROVERA PATIENTS WORKS!

- Discontinuation rates for DMPA users at 1 year are high in the absence of structured counseling: 70% in a New York study of low-income women *[Polaneczky-1996]*; 43.4% in a rural Mexican study *[Canto-DeCetina-2001]*
- Importance of focused, structured, repeated counseling at initiation and follow-up visits can't be overstated. See STRUCTURED COUNSELING p. 14
- Structured counseling may include repetition, having patient repeat back instructions, showing videotapes, providing videotapes, audiotapes and written instructions and asking focused questions such as "What has happened to your pattern of bleeding?", "Have your periods become extremely light?", OR "Does your pattern of bleeding bother you?" rather than unfocused questions like "Are you having any problems?"
- **Structured counseling in Mexico lowered DMPA discontinuation from three bleeding problems: amenorrhea, irregular bleeding and heavy bleeding, from 32% to 8%. Discontinuation from amenorrhea fell from 17 to 3%; from SPT or BTB from 10 to 3%; and from heavy bleeding from 5 to 2%** *[Canto-DeCetina-2001]*
- Weight should be taken at each visit and weight control discussed carefully if there has been weight gain (see progressive weight gain p. 129 and WEIGHT GAIN: A TEACHABLE MOMENT p. 132)

PROBLEM MANAGEMENT

Allergic reaction or vasovagal reaction: In acute setting, provide support as needed. Benadryl may reduce pruritus and swelling. Oxygen and other resuscitation may be needed for severe reactions (extremely rare). Most allergic manifestations subside in 1 week or so. Refer if symptoms severe or do not improve appropriately. Avoid future injections and help her choose a different method

Vaginal dryness (dyspareunia) or atrophic vaginitis: May be due to hypoestrogenism. Consider measuring E_2 levels and giving physiologic replacement dose of estrogen, if needed. May give estrogen as vaginal cream, ring, tablets or systemic estrogen (tablets or patch) supplementation. Dyspareunia may be relieved with water soluble or silicone lubricants

Pain or infection at injection site: Offer anti-inflammatory medications. Rule out infection or needle damage to nerve, etc. Provide appropriate antibiotics if infected.

Patient returns early (<11 weeks) wanting reinjection (eg b/c of travel): May give DMPA

Patient returns late (>13 weeks) for reinjection: See Figure 27.1 on page 135

Switching to another method (eg OCs, IUD, etc) from DMPA: Initiate new method at any time convenient for patient. Preferred time would be near end of effectiveness of last DMPA injection unless switching to OCs, patch or vaginal rings to control menstrual disorders on DMPA. **Do NOT wait until next menses to start pills.** She may have amenorrhea for a number of months after DMPA

Transitioning perimenopausal women: See Figure 27.2 on page 136

Weight gain: Advise to watch caloric intake and to increase exercise. Refer to OA, Overeaters Anonymous. **Be ready to discontinue method if weight gain is excessive or unacceptable** (See teachable moment p. 132)

Heavy bleeding:
- Rule out pregnancy, cervical infection or neoplasia and other causes
- Rule out anemia - recommend iron rich foods and/or supplements
- May treat with NSAIDs or low dose estrogen supplements:
  - Ibuprofen 800 mg orally every 8 hours for 3 days
  - Conjugated equine estrogen (2.5, 1.25 or 0.625 mg) orally once a day up to four times per day for 4-6 days OR ethinyl estradiol x 21 days (expensive)
  - COCs for 1-2 months (in addition to DMPA use)

Irregular bleeding and spotting:
- **Reassure that cumulative blood loss is usually less not more**
- Rule out infection or cervical lesions as source
- Reassure that irregular spotting and bleeding is to be expected in first several months
- May use same therapies as outlined in heavy bleeding section above

Amenorrhea:
- Reassure her that this is not a medical problem. Do pregnancy test if she has other Sx.
- Switch method if patient desires regular menses (consider patch, ring, COCs). Even if she stops DMPA, menses may not return for months

Depression:
- Evaluate suicide potential and refer immediately, if indicated. Patient should avoid alcohol
- Explain that DMPA usually does not worsen depression. Start antidepressant therapy, if needed. Discontinue DMPA if you or your patient has any misgivings about continuing its use

FERTILITY AFTER DISCONTINUATION OF METHOD
- **Because anovulation may last for more than 1 year, women who know they will want to become pregnant within one year of cessation of use would be wise to consider another option, especially women over 35 years of age**
- Average of 9-10 months delay to conception after last shot. (Delay not increased with increased duration of use). More than 90% of women become pregnant within 2 years
- Women who do not want to await spontaneous return of ovulation will require gonadotrophin therapy to induce ovulation. Gonadotropins will not overcome effect of DMPA on cervical mucus

Figure 27.1 Initial Injection or Late Reinjection (more than 13 and 0/7 weeks since last injection) of DMPA or Switching From DMPA to COCs or Another Hormonal Method*

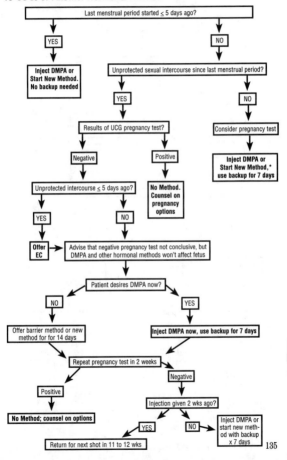

Figure 27.2 Making Transition from DMPA to Menopause, With or Without Hormone Replacement Therapy (HRT, EPT, or HT)

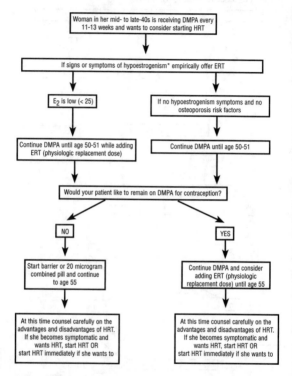

Woman in her mid- to late-40s is receiving DMPA every 11-13 weeks and wants to consider starting HRT

↓

If signs or symptoms of hypoestrogenism* empirically offer ERT

E₂ is low (< 25)

If no hypoestrogenism symptoms and no osteoporosis risk factors

Continue DMPA until age 50-51 while adding ERT (physiologic replacement dose)

Continue DMPA until age 50-51

Would your patient like to remain on DMPA for contraception?

NO

YES

Start barrier or 20 microgram combined pill and continue to age 55

Continue DMPA and consider adding ERT (physiologic replacement dose) until age 55

At this time counsel carefully on the advantages and disadvantages of HRT. If she becomes symptomatic and wants HRT, start HRT OR start HRT immediately if she wants to

At this time counsel carefully on the advantages and disadvantages of HRT. If she becomes symptomatic and wants HRT, start HRT OR start HRT immediately if she wants to

* DMPA can suppress gonadotropins, so measuring FSH or LH is not informative of menopausal state. DMPA use decreases endogenous estrogen levels. Long-term DMPA users in their 40s may benefit from estrogen supplementation. Kaunitz supplements long-term DMPA users in their 40s with 1.25 mg of conjugated estrogen (or equivalent drug). Arbitrarily, at age 55, each woman, if she wants to and understands the risks and benefits, can be switched to conventional HRT. This is easy and minimizes need for laboratory testing, addresses the bone density issue, contraception, and vasomotor concerns while maintaining amenorrhea. [Kaunitz, 1998]

IMPLANTS: IMPLANON – THE SINGLE ETONOGESTREL IMPLANT

DESCRIPTION: Single implant is 4-cm long and 2 mm in diameter (5 mm longer than one Norplant implant), with a membrane of ethylene vinyl acetate (EVA) copolymer and with a core of 68 mg of etonogestrel in EVA (the new name for 3-ketodesogestrel). Progestin released at rate of 60 µg per day. Implanon is effective for 3 years. Implant is placed under the skin of upper arm with a 19 gauge disposable, preloaded inserter

EFFECTIVENESS: No pregnancies in earliest studies. Some postmarketing pregnancies. Overall, 82% of women continue to use Implanon for 2 or more years

MECHANISM
- Within 24 hours of insertion thick cervical mucus prevents normal sperm transport
- Inhibition of ovulation. 0% in first 2 years and only 2 women, .6%, had 4 ovulatory events in third year of Implanon use
- Atrophic endometrium

COST: Not determined, but comparable to an IUD

ADVANTAGES
Menstrual: Decreased menstrual and ovulatory cramping or pain; overall, less bleeding than with Norplant and more amenorrhea (20% at one year). Less anemia. With the use of Implanon, uterine pain was reduced or eliminated in 88% of women previously experiencing dysmenorrhea [Affandi 1998]
Sexual/psychological:
- Sexual intercourse may be more pleasurable because fear of pregnancy is reduced
- Applied at time independent of sexual intercourse—allows spontaneity
Cancers/tumors and masses: None
Other:
- High continuation rate in clinical trials. Cyclic headaches may improve
- Single implant is easier and faster to insert and remove than multiple implants. Removal is usually accomplished with only a #11 scapel and gentle finger pressure with 0.1 ml of local anesthetic (use tuberculm syringe)
- Assymptomatic (usually) follicular cysts are less common than with Mirena or Norplant

DISADVANTAGES
Menstrual:
- Unpredictable/irregular menstrual bleeding frequent and may persist
- Amenorrhea and oligomenorrhea common
Sexual/psychological:
- Irregular bleeding may inhibit sexual intercourse
- Insertion and removal require procedures, for which special training is needed
Cancers/tumors and masses: None
Other:
- No STI protection
- Hormonal side effects: headache is most common
- May develop acne

COMPLICATIONS: Removal difficulties much less frequent than with Norplant

CANDIDATES FOR USE: ←

- Implanon is particularly good for women with contraindications to or side effects from estrogen:
  - Women with personal history of thrombosis
  - Recently postpartum women
  - Women who are exclusively breast-feeding
  - Smokers over age 35
  - Women who had or fear chloasma, worsening migraine headaches, hypertriglyceridemia or other estrogen-related side effects
  - Women with hypertension, coronary artery disease or cerebrovascular disease

PRESCRIBING PRECAUTIONS, MEDICAL ELIGIBILITY CHECKLIST, INITIATING METHOD: Same precautions as for progestin-only pills ←

INSTRUCTIONS FOR PATIENT: Irregular bleeding is to be expected and persists while rod is in place. If your pattern of bleeding is unacceptable, come back because there are several treatments that may make your bleeding pattern more acceptable. Amenorrhea more likely than with Norplant, but less likely than with DMPA

FOLLOW-UP: Routine GYN follow-up ←

PROBLEM MANAGEMENT: ←

Amenorrhea: Quite common. Pregnancy test if symptoms of pregnancy
Spotting/breakthrough bleeding: to be expected; not harmful. If bothersome may provide several cycles of lowo-dose pills, or NSAID
Arm Pain after insertion
- Rule out nerve damage or infection
- If due to bruising, advise her to make sure bandage is not too tight
- Apply ice packs for 24 hours
- Take acetaminophen or NSAID
Infection in insertion area
- *No abscess:* cellulitis only. Do not remove, Clean infected area with antiseptic. Oral antibiotics for 7 days. (Recheck in 24-48 hours and at end of therapy)
- *Abscess:* Preload with antibiotics; prepare infected area with antiseptic, make incision, drain pus, and remove implant. Continue antibiotic therapy and wound care
Difficult to locate rod: may be found by ultrasound, by mammography or MRI. This ← requires experienced sonographer using tranducer of 10 MHz or greater

FERTILITY AFTER DISCONTINUATION OF USE: Return to baseline fertility is rapid and complete; 94% ovulate within 3-6 weeks of removal

INSERTION TECHNIQUE: 6 TIPS ←

1. Be sure implant is in the inserter
2. Place local anesthetic (2 cc of 1% lidocaine) along 4 cm track, 6-8 cm above anticubital space on nondominant arm
3. Tent up skin to ensure **SUPERFICIAL INSERTION JUST UNDER SKIN.**
4. Introduce implant by pulling skin taut, introduce needle at 20° angle.
5. Break plastic seal by pressing the obturator support bar (rod or plunger). Flip support bar 90°. Stabilize obturator (inner rod) and withdraw outer needle over obturator. DO NOT PUSH OBTURATOR IN!!!
6. **MAKE SURE TO PALPATE AND, LATER, HAVE PATIENT PALPATE** to be sure contraceptive rod is in place. Pregnancies occur when there is no rod in a woman's arm!

IMPLANTS: JADELLE - 2 IMPLANTS

DESCRIPTION:
- Norplant II or Jadelle is very similar to Norplant but consists of 2 slightly larger "rods" rather than 6 "capsules"
- Actually has been approved as a 5-year contraceptive by U.S. FDA. Not yet marketed in U.S.
- 5-year contraceptive effectiveness rates documented (Sivin et al)

IMPLANTS: NORPLANT - 6 IMPLANTS

DESCRIPTION: 6 soft plastic (silastic) implants (34 mm in length and 2.4 mm in diameter) are inserted into the subcutaneous tissue beneath the skin of the medial aspect of a woman's non-dominant upper arm. Each implant is filled with 36 mg of levonorgestrel powder, which is slowly released through micropores in the implant to achieve an average plasma concentration of 0.30 ng/ml over 5 years. Since Norplant is not currently available, much of the information on this excellent method has been left out of this edition (See the 2000-2001 edition of ***Managing Contraception***). As of March 2003, there are no plans for Norplant to be reintroduced in the U.S. For more information: ***www.popcouncil.org*** or ***www.wyeth.com/news***. The latest data show that the last Norplant lot, which was recalled due to concerns about efficacy, actually is effective. Women no longer have to use backup as was previously recommended (from Wyeth bulletin).

EFFECTIVENESS *[Trussell J IN Contraceptive Technology-18th edition]*
- Product labeling indicates the system is effective for up to 5 years. Is effective for 7 years or more in women ≤ 154 pounds or women over age 35

Perfect use failure rate in first year: 0.05% (1 woman in 2,000)

Typical use failure rate in first year: 0.05%

Cumulative 7 year failure rate: 1.9% *[Contraception 61:187, 2000]*

(failure rate higher beyond 5 years in obese women (>90 kg or 200 pounds);
recommend back up if leaving implants in for contraception beyond 5 years in women weighing 200 pounds or more)

For further information on Norplant, see past editions of this book and Contraceptive Technology
Contact your Wyeth rep if you cannot find someone to remove a patient's implants

CHAPTER 28

Female Sterilization: Tubal Ligation or Occlusion

DESCRIPTION: Surgery to interrupt the patency of fallopian tubes. In 1995 in the USA, 24% of married women reported having had tubal sterilization while 15% of their husbands had had a vasectomy. *[Chandra, 1998]* Many tubal sterilizations are performed on single women. Approximately half of sterilizations in the USA are done in the immediate postpartum period within 48 hours of delivery *[Peterson, 1998]*.

EFFECTIVENESS

Failure rates differ by sterilization method and patient's age. Data for transcervical methods (ESSURE) (see p. 144) are available for only 3 years of follow up (0% at 3 years)

Table 28.1 Cumulative 10-year failure rates for some methods of voluntary female sterilization methods*

Method	Failure rate (highest rate)	
Postpartum partial salpingectomy	0.8%*	For each sterilization method, at least 50% more failures were ascertained AFTER 2 YEARS as had been identified in the 2 years immediately following the sterilization procedure
Silastic bands over loop of tube	1.8%*	
Interval partial salpingectomy	2.0%*	
Bipolar cautery	2.5%*	
Spring clip application	3.7%*	
Filshie clip (7 years)	0.9%+	

* U.S. Collaborative Review of Sterilization. The risk of pregnancy after tubal sterilization. Am J Obstet Gynecol 1996;174:1161-70.

+ Filshie clip (0.9% failure rate - 7 years) [Chi-Chen Contraception 1987;35:171-8]

- Younger women had higher failure rates
- All methods require proper application to maximize effectiveness
- Teaching institution rates(above study) may differ from private settings

MECHANISM: Interruption of patency of the fallopian tubes preferably in isthmic region thereby preventing fertilization

LAPAROSCOPIC STERILIZATION: TRANSABDOMINAL

Bipolar cautery:
- Apply to area along fallopian tube with no vessels ascending through broad ligament, where the diameter of tube similar on either side of damaged area (at least 2 cm from uterotubal junction). Thoroughly cauterize tissue using bipolar cutting current of 25 Watts passes through jaws of instrument. Bipolar cautery has the highest risk of subsequent fistulization and ectopic pregnancy.

Silastic band: (Fallope ring, Yoon band)
- Apply over knuckle of tube at least 3 cm from utero-tubal junction. Loop of tube clearly contain two complete ligaments of tube

Hulka-Clemens clip (spring clip):
- Spring-loaded clip. Apply to isthmic portion of tube. 1-2 cm distal to cornu at an angle of 90% relative to long axis of tube. Highest failure rate

Filshie clip:
- Hinged titanium clip with cured silicone rubber lining. Apply to isthmic portion of tube, 1 to 2 cm from cornu. Should see hook end of clip through filmy mesosalpinx. May apply ◄ postpartum with special applicator (0.9% failure vs. 0.27% failure for interval application)

140

Figure 28.1 Laparoscopic Technique Diagrams

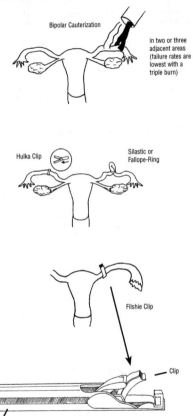

Bipolar Cauterization

in two or three adjacent areas (failure rates are lowest with a triple burn)

Hulka Clip

Silastic or Fallope-Ring

Filshie Clip

Clip

Applicator

Filshie Clip (enlarged, in applicator)

POSTPARTUM OR INTERVAL MINI-LAPAROTOMY METHODS

Modified Pomeroy:
- Ligation at the base of a loop of isthmic portion of tube with plain absorbable catgut suture (tied twice) followed by excision of the knuckle of tube

Modified Parkland:
- Excision of segment of isthmic portion of tube after separate ligation of cut ends

Irving:
- Doubly ligate and sever tube. Bury proximal stump into uterus and put distal stump into mesosalpinx. Poor potential for reversal and higher risk of intraoperative bleeding

Uchida:
- Inject mesenteric part of tube with saline. Divide muscular part of tube/excise 3-5 cm. Bury proximal tube and exteriorize or excise distal tube. Poor potential for reversal

Fimbriectomy:
- Excision of fimbria of tube. Poor potential for reversal

Figure 28.2 Postpartum or Mini-Laparotomy Techniques

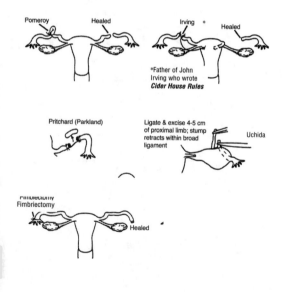

Pomeroy   Healed

Irving *   Healed

*Father of John
Irving who wrote
Cider House Rules

Pritchard (Parkland)

Ligate & excise 4-5 cm
of proximal limb; stump
retracts within broad
ligament   Uchida

Fimbriectomy
Fimbriectomy   Healed

ADVANTAGES

Menstrual: None

Sexual/psychological: Enhanced enjoyment of sex by reducing worry of pregnancy

Cancers, tumors, and masses:
- Decreased risk of ovarian cancer. Women with BRCA 1 mutations who have undergone a tubal ligation have a 60% lower risk of developing invasive ovarian cancer. *[Narod-Lancet 357 (9267): 1467-70, 2001]*

Other:
- Permanent and highly effective

DISADVANTAGES

Menstrual:
- Data from 9514 women who underwent tubal sterilization by 6 techniques and followed for up to 5 years suggest no "post-tubal ligation syndrome" and no increases in the amount or duration of menstrual bleeding or menstrual pain. *[Peterson, 2000]*

Sexual/psychological:
- Regret may occur especially with young patients; counsel well and offer reversible methods if any hesitancy (see Fig. 28.5, p. 146)

Cancers, tumors, and masses: None

Other:
- Requires outpatient surgery (usually with general anesthesia); Expensive in short term
- If failure occurs, higher risk of ectopic pregnancy (10%-65%)
- Not readily reversible and does not prevent spread of HIV and STIs

COMPLICATIONS *[Peterson, 1997]*

	Minilaparotomy	Laparoscopy
Minor	11.6%	6.0%
Major	1.5%	0.9%

- Minor complications include infection, wound separation
- Major complications include conversion to laparotomy, hemorrhage, viscus injury especially with cautery, anesthetic complications
- Major vessel injury risk with laparoscopy 3-9/10,000 procedures
- Mortality: 1-2/100,000 procedures (leading cause is general anesthesia)

LONG-TERM RISKS

- Statistically higher risk for subsequent hysterectomy, but only in women who had gynecologic complaints prior to sterilization
- Regret (0.9% - 26.0%) Risk factors include: age under 30, low parity, sterilization at time of cearean section, change in marital status, poverty, minority status, misinformation about permanence or risks, decision made in a hurry. The risk of regret is 40% at 14 years in women having tubal sterilization under 30. **This issue requires careful counseling**

CANDIDATES FOR USE

- Woman who is certain she wants no more children
- Woman over age 21 (only required for Medicaid reimbursement, not for medical requirements or for California state funding)
- Woman for whom surgery is considered safe

Adolescents: Not a preferred method, generally higher regret and higher failure rates

ESSURE: HYSTEROSCOPIC STERILIZATION VIA POLYESTER FIBERS

www.essure.com Essure is a new approach to transcervical sterilization that causes tubal blockage by encouraging local tissue growth with polyesther (PET) fibers *[Valle Fertil Steril 2001]*. An attached outer coiled spring is released that molds to the shape of the interstitial (uterine) portion of each fallopian tube. The device costs $950 *[Ballagh, 2003]*, but it is covered by insurance plans that cover laparoscopic tubal ligation (even Medicaid). It takes 3 months after procedure to occlude tubes. An hysterosaplingogram (HSG) is needed 3 months after surgery to document success

Figure 28.3 Essure System Overview: Micro-Insert Design

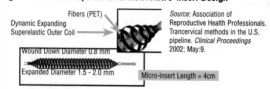

Fibers (PET)
Dynamic Expanding Superelastic Outer Coil

Wound Down Diameter 0.8 mm
Expanded Diameter 1.5 - 2.0 mm

Micro-insert Length = 4cm

Source: Association of Reproductive Health Professionals. Trancervical methods in the U.S. pipeline. *Clinical Proceedings* 2002; May:9.

ADVANTAGES "The alternative to incision"

• Provides tubal sterilization in physician's or ambulatory surgery office (average operating time: 13 to 35 minutes)
• It is the woman's own tissue plus the implant that causes tubal occlusion
• No major change in a woman's menstrual cycles
• No failures among 453 women relying on Essure for one year following confirmation of tubal blockage at 3 months by hysteroscopy; 99.8% effective @ 2 years
• There is no need for conscious sedation or general anesthesia (nonsteriodal premedication is strongly recommended to prevent tubal spasm)
• In clinical trial, (Australia, Europe, and the U.S.) 92% of women returned to work in one day, most resumed normal activities the same day as the procedure
• May be preferred for obese women, women with abdominal adhesions, or women with risk factors for anesthesia

DISADVANTAGES: Requires specialized training and equipment

• Hysterosaplingogram must be done at 3 months to confirm blockage. Until that time, couple must use another contraceptive.
• Procedure designed for interval sterilization. It is not to be used at Cesarean section or immediately postpartum *[Bullagh, 2003]*
• Luteal pregnancies occured in 4 of 466 women in spite of negative urine pregnancy tests on the day of the procedure
• It may not be possible to visualize both tubal ostia (this occurs about 2% of the time)
• May require more than one operative procedure
• In only 446 of 518 women (86.1%) could devices be introduced into both tubes at the time of the first procedure due to lateral tubes, tubal spasm or tube already not patent
• Tubal spasm may occur
• Expulsion of one or both devices (14 of 466 successful procedures or 3.0%)
• Perforation of the uterus occured during 4 of 466 procedures
• This form of sterilization cannot be reversed

PRESTERILIZATION COUNSELING CHECKLIST*

- Discuss alternative reversible methods and quote their effectiveness. (IUDs and implants are more effective than some forms of tubal sterilization)
- Discuss vasectomy as an alternative
- Insure patient commitment to having no future children, even if something happened to her current family
- Describe details of surgery (informed consent later) and possible intraoperative and long-term complications (risk for ectopic pregnancy)
- Stress that procedure must be considered irreversible and that about 10% of women regret their decision and answer all of her questions
- Obtain informed consent using locally approved consent forms - No requirement that spouse must be involved

*Adapted from ACOG Technical Bulletin, April 1996.

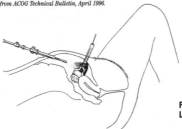

**Figure 28.4
Laparoscopy**

INITIATING METHOD

- Obtain informed consent. Preferable to involve partner in process, but not necessary
- Any time in cycle with certainty of no conception, otherwise follicular timing preferred
- The routine provision of antibiotics is generally NOT recommended *[see ACOG Practice Bulletin No. 23, January 2001]*

FOLLOW-UP

- For women having interval occlusion procedure, follow up in two weeks for post-op wound check can be performed, but not necessary. Routine annual gynecology exams
- 3-month follow up visit for Essure (see p. 140)

MANAGEMENT OF PROBLEMS

- Anesthesia complications, wound infections, intraperitoneal adhesion formation, hydrosalpinx – managed with standard tools
- Although some women report irregular menses or dysmenorrhea after tubal sterilization, several studies have demonstrated that a syndrome of irregular menses or dysmenorrhea following tubal sterilization does NOT exist *[Peterson-2000]*. These problems are **not** apt to develop at any higher rates in sterilized women. They are most likely age-related and inevitable

FERTILITY AFTER TUBAL STERILIZATION

- Women must desire to be permanently sterile because reversal is costly and results are unpredictable. In vitro fertilization may be possible, but many cannot afford this procedure and it is not always successful

Figure 28.5 Sterilization Requested by Young Woman

Woman in early 20's seeking tubal sterilization after 2-3 children

↓

Inform her that vasectomy is safer, extremely effective and more easily reversed

↓

Inform her that risk of regret following tubal sterilization is higher in the United States if she is:
- Young
- Unmarried (single, separated or divorced)
- Unmarried now but is married later on, especially if new husband wants a child with her
- Married now but becomes divorced later
- On Medicaid or has a very low or no income
- African-American or Hispanic
- Close to the end of a pregnancy (postpartum, post-therapeutic abortion or post-miscarriage)
- Thinking that tubal sterilization is easy to reverse (it is both very expensive and about 60% effective). Essure, the new transcervical sterilization technique, is particularly difficult to reverse. More often now in-vitro fertilization is attempted. It is very expensive and may not be successful

↓

- Encourage her to consider waiting until her later 20's or early 30's for tubal sterilization
- Encourage use of effective long-term contraceptive: Copper T 380 A or Levonorgestrel IUD (Mirena)
- In encouraging her to delay sterilization, use gentle encouragement not strong-arm tactics
- Be sure she knows that the final decision is *hers* to make, not yours

↓

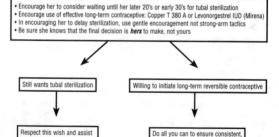

Still wants tubal sterilization

↓

Respect this wish and assist her in accomplishing her goal

Willing to initiate long-term reversible contraceptive

↓

Do all you can to ensure consistent, correct use of reversible method. Remain willing to provide her with sterilization at her request

DESCRIPTION: Permanent male contraception. Outpatient surgical procedure. No-scalpel technique punctures scrotum, delivers vas; ligates or cauterizes vas. Nearly 1 in 5 white U.S. men married to women of childbearing age has had a vasectomy. *[Amba-1997]*

EFFECTIVENESS (See Table 13.2, p. 39)
Perfect use failure rate in first year: 0.10%
Typical use failure rate in first year: 0.15%
[Trussell J, IN Contraceptive Technology, 2004]

Although vasectomy is safer and potentially more effective than tubal sterilization, as of mid-2000, there are only 4 nations in the world where vasectomies exceed tubal sterilizations: Great Britain, the Netherlands, New Zealand and Bhutan.

Recent analysis of the 540 women in the CREST study who were protected by vasectomy found a cumulative failure rate of 9.4 per 1000 procedures at one year (0.9%) and 11.3 at years 2, 3 and 5. *[Jamieson, Costello, Trussell et al-2004]*

MECHANISM

Interrupts vas deferens preventing passage of sperm into seminal fluid and female reproductive tract

Vas deferens isolated following incision with scalpel

ADVANTAGES

Sexual/psychological:
- Sexual intercourse may be more enjoyable because fear of pregnancy decreased
- Permits man opportunity to take on an important contraceptive role
- No interference during sexual intercourse and no contraceptive burden for female

Cancers, tumors, and masses: None

Other:
- Simpler, safer and more effective than female sterilization
- More cost-effective than female sterilization and more convenient
- Shares contraception responsibility with partner
- No supplies or further clinic visits needed after sperm count has been documented to be zero
- General anesthesia rarely required

DISADVANTAGES

Sexual/ psychological:
- Some men resist vasectomy fearing that it will interfere with sexual function (it doesn't) or because they feel contraception is solely the woman's responsibility (it isn't)
- Regret at a later time possible (1% of men request a reversal)
- Will need back-up method until there are no motile sperm. Female partner may still ◄ need contraception if she has other partner(s) or if STI protection needed

Cancers, tumors, and masses: None

Other:
- Does not reduce risk for STIs; will still need to use condom if at risk
- Short-term post-operative discomfort, bruising, and swelling

COMPLICATIONS

- Surgically related complaints such as hematoma, bruising, wound infection, or adverse reaction to local anesthesia
- Severe chronic pain (2%) *[Choe, Kirkema - 1996]*. Usually limited to less than 1 year
- Later regret possible

CANDIDATES FOR USE: Men who desire a permanent method

INITIATING METHOD
- Take preoperative history; make general health assessment
- Ask if history of genital problems
- Obtain informed consent. In general, try to involve partner
- Carefully counsel, especially about permanence of method
- Advise patient to bathe genital area and upper thighs prior to surgery; wear clean, loose-fitting clothes to facility; no food for 2 hours before procedure

PRESCRIBING PRECAUTIONS
- Current infection of penis, prostate, or scrotum
- Fear of needles or scalpels (scalpels not required if no-scalpel vasectomy)

INSTRUCTIONS FOR PATIENT
- Plan to rest for 48 hours
- Apply ice pack to incision site to decrease swelling, pain and bruising. Small packages of frozen peas conform well around the scrotum
- Keep area dry for two days – wear snug underwear and pants to provide support where needed
- If any symptoms or signs of infection develop, seek help immediately.
- Return as directed for sperm counts. Results from a new study suggest that azospermia is more likely after 12 weeks (60% azospermia) than after 20 ejaculations (28% azospermic) and that neither endpoint is ideal *[Barone-2003]*. Use other forms of contraception until two consecutive sperm samples show no motile sperm

FOLLOW-UP: *To avoid failure due to LATE recanalization, repeating semen analysis every few years makes sense*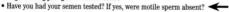
- Have you had your semen tested? If yes, were motile sperm absent?

PROBLEM MANAGEMENT
Wound infection: Treat with antibiotics. Drain and treat any abscesses
Hematoma: Apply warm moist packs to scrotum. Provide scrotal support
Granuloma: Observe; usually it will resolve itself. Occasionally requires surgery
Pain at site: If no infection, provide scrotal support and analgesics
Excessive swelling: If large and painful, may require surgery. Provide scrotal support if hematoma
Chronic persistent pain considered to be severe: [2% - Choe, Kirkema - 1996]. IPPF Handbook states that this pain can often be relieved by vasovasectomy or decompression of the distended vas deferens releasing the sperm into the scrotal cavity *[Evans, Huezo IPPF Handbook - 1997]*

FERTILITY AFTER VASECTOMY
- Man must accept that vasectomy is irreversible and permanent
- Microsurgical techniques of reversal now result in return of sperm to ejaculate in over 90% of men, but in pregnancy rates of only 50% or above. Reversibility rates decrease as time since procedure increases
- Important factors for reversal are
  - skill of microsurgeon
  - length of time from vasectomy
  - presence of antisperm antibodies (man)
  - partner's fertility
  - manner in which vasectomy was performed (amount of vas removed or cauterized)

Figure 29.1 Vasectomy – No-Scalpel Techniques

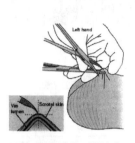

A) Piercing the skin with the medial blade of the dissecting forceps

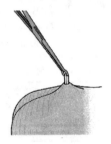

B) Grasping a partial thickness of the elevated vas at the crest of the loop, with only the ringed clamp attached

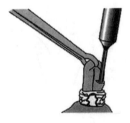

Cautery with a blunt wire inserted into the hemitransected vas (done in each direction)

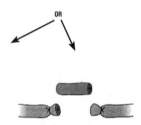

OR

Ligation and section

Cornell No-Scalpel Vasectomy Center. No-Scalpel Vasectomy. http://www.vasectomy.com/no-scalpel-vasectomy-diagram.html.2/6/02.

CHAPTER 30

Future Methods

www.popcouncil.org or www.conrad.org OR www.plannedparenthood.org
/ARTICLES/bcfuture-w.html

NEW HORMONAL FORMULATIONS FOR ORAL USE
• Several lower-dose COCs are currently available in Europe with 15 µg of EE

Table 30.1 PROGESTIN-ONLY IMPLANTS

NAME	# CAPSULES	HORMONE	LENGTH OF USE	BIODEGRADABLE
Norplant 2	2	Levonorgestrel	5 yrs.	no
Uniplant	1	nomegestrol		no
Nestorone	1	nestorone	2 yrs.	no
Implanon	1	etonogestrel	3 yrs.	no
Annuelle	pellets	norethindrone		yes

VAGINAL DELIVERY SYSTEMS
• Progestin-only vaginal rings: may be worn continuously and last up to a year ◄——
  NOTE: Contraceptive vaginal rings that release only a progestin have been studied. Like other progestin-only methods, however, they have a slightly lower effectiveness and slightly higher rates of spotting and bleeding between menses. Progestin-only rings may prove in the future to be a good option for women who are postpartum or breastfeeding or who have contraindications to estrogen containing methods.
• Progesterone daily suppositories

INTRAUTERINE DEVICES
• Gynefix Copper IUD: 6 sleeves of copper on a string that has one end embedded in fundus and other end protruding through cervix for monthly monitoring. IUD has low expulsion rate and cumulative 3-year failure rate of 0.5% (popular in Europe)
• Fibroplant: progestin-releasing fiber that is fixed in uterine wall

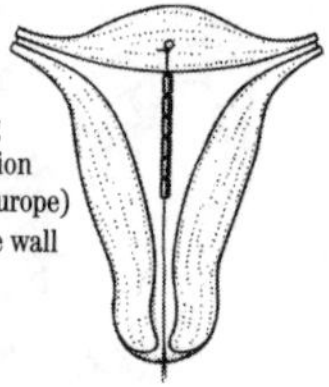

FEMALE BARRIERS
• New prototypes of female condoms
• Trials beginning on diaphragms that can be fitted by the woman instead of by her clinician
• Protectaid: new vaginal sponges

**Figure 30.2
Gynefix intrauterine
copper IUD**

MICROBICIDES
• Microbicides are entering effectiveness trials ◄——
• A microbicide is unlikely to reach the market until after 2010 ◄——

MALE METHODS
• Male hormonal methods under development often use exogenous progestin or gonadotropin-releasing hormone (GnRH) antagonist to suppress FSH and LH, thereby decreasing spermatogenesis. Replacement testosterone provided
  injectables: progestin + testosterone / GnRH + testosterone
  implants: 2 implant system with GnRH + androgen

- Testosterone (injectable, patch or implant) combined with slow release progestin implant
- Immunocontraception: Methods based on interference of the reproductive process by products of an immune reaction
- "Temporary sterilization"— injecting the vas deferens with a polymer to block sperm
- Anti-sperm compounds, e.g., gossypol from cottonseed oil and Triptolide

NEW EC METHODS: A variety will arise in the future; mifepristone, 10 mg, is effective

VACCINES: In phase 1 trials

QUINACRINE STERILIZATION (QS): Research on Quinacrine sterilization continues, but the method has been marred by controversy and bitter debate. The International Journal of Gynecology & Obstetrics, the official publication of FIGO, The International Federation of Gynecology and Obstetrics, (website: http://www.elsevier.com/locate/ijgo) has published an extensive supplement on 40,252 cases of Quinacrine sterilization. This 150 page document is edited by Dr. Jack Lippes, a longtime advocate of research on this approach to sterilization.

Quinacrine sterilization involves insertion of 7 pellets containing a total of 252 mg of quinacrine into the uterine cavity. This is repeated in one month (2 insertions of 252 mg of quinacrine each through an inserter very much like the inserter used for IUD insertion). In some protocols there are 3 insertions of quinacrine in this manner.

Lippes concludes "Results of clinical research reported in this Supplement are reassuring: the method seems safe, effective and simple enough not to require senior physicians for success." In fact, Lippes points out that in one study "The crude reported pregnancy rate for assistant doctors and midwives was lower than that for senior doctors (3.0 versus 5.5%)." Acceptability of QS is high "When QS is offered simultaneously with surgical sterilization, QS is preferred ten to one over surgical techniques."

Although questions about the efficacy of QS remain, Lippes notes that "It is clear now that QS is safer than tubectomy and even vasectomy as performed in Vietnam." Hieu, describing an early retrospective study of 15,190 users of tubectomy, QS and vasectomy in 5 provinces of Vietnam, found all 3 methods to be safe although morbidity associated with tubectomy was more serious than with QS or vasectomy. The failure rate was 1.0% for tubectomy, 4.1% with vasectomy and **13.2% with QS**, although only a small fraction of the QS failures were confirmed. Higher than expected pregnancies in this Vietnam field trial was due to "readily available menstrual regulation procedures, without confirmation of pregnancy. This was felt to be important because delayed menses is a common side effect of QS."

In the 2003 FIGO Supplement Zipper (Santiago, Chile) and Kessel (Portland, Oregon) conclude that "The original QS research in Chile continues to grow and it has been joined by a wide international population. QS safety is thoroughly demonstrated in long-term clinical experience in a wide variety of settings. **There is a growing consensus that the method should be made available to women where surgical sterilization is difficult to provide safely.** Prospects for improved efficacy matching that of surgical sterilization appear likely. Final approval by the US FDA of QS is now the highest priority for contraceptive development."

CHAPTER 31

Sexually Transmissible Infections (STIs)
2002 CDC Guidelines for Treatment*

Complete guidelines at www.cdc.gov/nchstp/od/nchstp.html
www.hab.hrsa.gov   www.aidsinfo.nih.gov

Since women and men seeking contraceptives are also at risk for STIs, we have included in this book information on the treatment of many of the most important STIs based on the latest CDC recommendations (2002).

CLINICAL PREVENTION GUIDELINES

• The specific recommendations presented here are from that document
• Both partners should get tested for STIs, including HIV, before initiating sexual intercourse
• A new condom should be used for each act of insertive intercourse (oral, vaginal or anal)

Prevention Methods
• **Male Condoms**
  • Used consistently and correctly, latex condoms are effective in preventing the transmission of HIV infection and can reduce the risk for other STIs
  • Failure usually results from inconsistent or incorrect use, rather than condom breakage

• **Female Condoms**
  • Laboratory studies indicate that the Reality female condom is an effective mechanical barrier to viruses, including HIV
  • Used consistently and correctly, the female condom may substantially reduce risk for STIs including HIV

• **Condoms and Spermicides**
  • Whether condoms used with vaginal application of spermicide are more effective than condoms used without vaginal spermicides has not been determined
  • Therefore, the consistent use of condoms, with or without spermicidal lubricant or vaginal application of spermicide, is recommended

* *Next anticipated CDC guidelines: 2006* ⬅

- However, vaginal spermicides containing N-9 are not effective in preventing cervical gonorrhea, chlamydia or HIV infection
- Diaphragm use has been demonstrated to provide some protection against cervical gonorrhea, chlamydia, and trichomoniasis (case control, cross sectional studies)
- Vaginal sponges or diaphragms should not be relied upon to protect women against HIV infection

- *Nonbarrier Contraception, Surgical Sterilization, and Hysterectomy*
  - Hormonal contraception (e.g., oral contraceptives, Norplant, and Depo-Provera) offer no protection against HIV or other STDs
  - Women who use hormonal or intrauterine contraception, have been surgically sterilized, or have had hysterectomies should still be counseled on the use of condoms for HIV/STI protection

SPECIAL POPULATIONS

Pregnant Women

- *Recommended Screening Tests*
  - Syphilis: all pregnant women at first prenatal visit; high risk (high areas of syphilis morbidity) retested in early third trimester and at delivery
  - Hepatitis B surface antigen (HbsAg): all pregnant women first visit
  - *Neisseria gonorrhoeae*: first visit for women at risk or living in an area of high prevalence
  - *Chlamydia trachomatis*: at first prenatal visit and in the third trimester for women at increased risk (i.e., women aged <25 years and women who have a new or more than one sex partner or whose partner has other partners)
  - HIV screening test: encouraged for all pregnant women as routine prenatal test at the first prenatal visit
  - Bacterial vaginosis (BV): may be performed at the first prenatal visit for patients at high risk for preterm labor (history of prematurity). Current evidence does not support universal testing for BV
  - Papanicolaou (Pap) smear: first visit if no Pap smear has been documented during the preceding year
  - Hepatitis C antibodies should be performed at the first prenatal visit for women at high risk (intravenous drug users, blood transfusions, organ transplant)

- *Other Concerns (Other STI-related Concerns are to Be Considered as Follows:)*
  - Pregnant women who have either primary genital herpes infection, HBV, primary cytomegalovirus (CMV) infection, or Group B streptococcal infection and women who have syphilis and who are allergic to penicillin may need to be referred to an expert for management
  - HbsAg-positive pregnant women should be reported to the local and/or state health department; household and sexual contacts of HbsAg-positive women should be tested and immunized if negative
  - In the absence of lesions during the third trimester, routine serial culture for herpes simplex virus (HSV) is not indicated for women who have a history of recurrent genital herpes. However, obtaining cultures from such women at the time of delivery may be useful in guiding neonatal management. Prophylactic cesarean section is not indicated for women who do not have active genital lesions at the time of delivery
  - The presence of genital warts is not an indication for cesarean section unless size obstructs delivery in labor (rare)

Adolescents

- With limited exceptions, all U.S. adolescents can consent to the confidential diagnosis and treatment of STIs. See Table 6.1, p. 19

DISEASES CHARACTERIZED BY GENITAL ULCERS

Management of Patients Who Have Genital Ulcers
- In the United States, most young, sexually active patients who have genital ulcers have genital herpes, a smaller percentage have syphilis, or chancroid. Each disease has been associated with an increased risk for HIV infection
- The evaluation of all patients who have genital ulcers should include a serologic test for syphilis and diagnostic evaluation for herpes; in settings where chancroid is prevalent a test for *Haemophilis ducreyi* should be performed. Specific tests (to be used with clinical assessment) for the evaluation of genital ulcers include the following:
  - Serology, dark-field exam or direct immunofluorescence test for *T. pallidum*
  - Culture or antigen test for HSV and
  - Culture for *Haemophilus ducreyi*
- HIV testing should be a) performed in the management of patients who have genital ulcers caused by *T. pallidum* or *H. ducreyi* and b) considered for those who have ulcers caused by HSV

CHANCROID (SHAN-kroyd)

Organism: H. ducreyi

Diagnosis: Culture on special medium of *H. ducreyi*, or if the following criteria are met:
a) patient has 1 or more ulcers; b) no evidence of syphilis on lab exam after at least 7 days;
c) the clinical picture is typical of chancroid and d) test for HSV is negative.

Treatment: Recommended Regimens

Azithromycin	1 g orally in a single dose, OR
Ceftriaxone	250 mg intramuscularly (IM) in a single dose, OR
Ciprofloxacin	500 mg orally twice a day for 3 days, OR
Erythromycin base	500 mg orally three times a day for 7 days.

Follow-up: Re-examine in 3-7 days. If no improvement consider whether a) the diagnosis is correct, b) the patient is coinfected with another STI, c)the patient is infected with HIV, d) the treatment was not taken as instructed, or e) the *H. ducreyi* strain causing the infection is resistant to the prescribed antimicrobial.

- *The time required for complete healing*
  - Depends on the size of the ulcer; large ulcers may require >2 weeks
  - Healing is slower for some uncircumcised men who have ulcers under the foreskin
  - Resolution of fluctuant lymphadenopathy is slower than that of ulcers and may require drainage, even during otherwise successful therapy
  - Although needle aspiration of buboes is a simple procedure, incision and drainage of buboes may be preferred because of less need for subsequent drainage procedures

Management of Sex Partners: Should be examined and treated regardless of symptoms if they had sexual contact within 10 days of the onset of symptoms

Special Considerations: Pregnancy. The safety of azithromycin for pregnant and lactating women has not been established. Ciprofloxacin is contraindicated during pregnancy. No adverse effects of chancroid on pregnancy outcome or on the fetus have been reported.

GENITAL HERPES SIMPLEX VIRAL (HSV) INFECTION (Her-pes)

Most persons shed the virus intermittently and are unaware that they are infected and are asymptomatic at the time of transmission.
Organisms: HSV-1 and HSV-2
Diagnosis: See complete *2002 CDC Guidelines* or *Contraceptive Technology (18th Edition)*

Counseling: Counseling of these patients should include the following:

- Patients should be advised to abstain from sexual activity when lesions or prodromal symptoms are present and encouraged to inform their sex partners
- Latex condoms, when used consistently and correctly, can reduce the risk for genital herpes, when the infected areas are covered or protected by the condom
- Sexual transmission of HSV can occur during asymptomatic periods
- The risk for neonatal infection should be explained to all patients, including men. Childbearing-aged women who have genital herpes should be advised to inform health-care providers who care for them during pregnancy about the HSV infection
- Patients having a first episode of genital herpes should be advised that a) episodic antiviral therapy during recurrent episodes might shorten the duration of lesions and b) suppressive antiviral therapy can ameliorate or prevent recurrent outbreaks

Treatment: 5% to 30% of first-episode cases of genital herpes are caused by HSV-1, but clinical recurrences are much less frequent for HSV-1 than HSV-2 genital infection

---

- ***HSV, Recommended Regimens for First Clinical Infection***

Acyclovir	400 mg orally three times a day for 7-10 days, OR
Acyclovir	200 mg orally five times a day for 7-10 days, OR
Famciclovir	250 mg orally three times a day for 7-10 days, OR
Valacyclovir	1.0 g orally twice a day for 7-10 days

- ***HSV, Recommended Regimens for Episodic Recurrent Infection***

Acyclovir	400 mg orally three times a day for 5 days, OR
Acyclovir	200 mg orally five times a day for 5 days, OR
Acyclovir	800 mg orally twice a day for 5 days, OR
Famciclovir	125 mg orally twice a day for 5 days, OR
Valacyclovir	500 mg orally twice a day for 3-5 days, OR
Valacyclovir	1.0 g orally once a day for 5 days

- ***HSV, Recommended Regimens for Daily Suppressive Therapy***

Acyclovir	400 mg orally twice a day, OR
Famciclovir	250 mg orally twice a day, OR
Valacyclovir	250 mg orally twice a day, OR
Valacyclovir	500 mg orally once a day

- Valacyclovir 500 mg once a day appears less effective than other valacyclovir dosing regimens in patients who have very frequent recurrences (i.e., >10 episodes per year)
- Valacyclovir and famciclovir appear to be comparable to acyclovir in clinical outcome
- However, valacyclovir and famciclovir may be easier to take

Severe Disease: IV therapy should be provided for patients who have severe disease or complications necessitating hospitalization, such as disseminated infection, pneumonitis, hepatitis, or complications of the central nervous system (e.g., meningitis or encephalitis)

- ***HSV, Recommended Regimen for Persons with Severe Disease***

Acyclovir	5-10 mg/kg body weight IV every 8 hours for 5-7 days until clinical resolution is attained

---

Special Considerations:

- Pregnancy
  - Available data do not indicate an increased risk for major birth defects in women treated with acyclovir in the first trimester
  - Safety of valacyclovir, and famciclovir Rx in pregnant women not established

- *Perinatal Infection*
  - The risk for transmission to the neonate from an infected mother is high (30% - 50%) among women who acquire genital herpes near the time of delivery and is low (3%) among women who have a history of recurrent herpes at term and women who acquire genital HSV during the first half of pregnancy
  - Therefore, prevention of neonatal herpes should emphasize prevention of acquisition of genital HSV infection during late pregnancy
  - Susceptible women whose partners have oral or genital HSV infection, or those whose sex partners' infection status is unknown, should be counseled to avoid unprotected genital and oral sexual contact during late pregnancy
  - The results of viral cultures during pregnancy do not predict viral shedding at the time of delivery, and such cultures are not indicated routinely
  - At the onset of labor, all women should be examined and carefully questioned about whether they have symptoms of HSV. Infants of women who do not have symptoms or signs of HSV infection or its prodrome may be delivered vaginally
  - Cesarean delivery does not completely eliminate the risk for HSV infection in the neonate

GRANULOMA INGUINALE (DONOVANOSIS) (gran-u-LO-ma in-gwi-NAL-e, don-o-van-O-sis)

Organism: Calymmatobacterium granulomatis is an intracellular, gram-negative bacterium. It is seen rarely in the USA. Presents as a painless, progressive, vascular, ulcerative lesion with regional lymphadenopathy.

Diagnosis: Visualization of Donovan bodies from tissue of lesion

Treatment: Appears to halt progressive destruction of tissue. Prolonged duration of therapy often required to enable granulation and re-epithelialization of the ulcers. Therapy should be continued until all lesions have healed completely

- *Granuloma Inguinale, Recommended Regimens*

Doxycycline..............................100 mg orally twice a day for a minimum of 3 weeks
Trimethoprim-
sulfamethoxazole...................One double-strength tablet orally twice a day for a minimum
of 3 weeks, OR

- *Granuloma Inguinale, Alternative Regimens*

Ciprofloxacin..........................750 mg orally twice a day for a minimum of 3 weeks, OR
Erythromycin base.................500 mg orally four times a day for a minimum of 3 weeks
(for use during pregnancy), OR
Azithromycin.............................1 g orally per week for at least 3 weeks

NOTE: For any of the above regimens, the addition of an aminoglycoside (gentamicin 1 mg/kg IV every 8 hours) should be considered if lesions do not respond within the first few days of therapy

LYMPHOGRANULOMA VENEREUM (LGV) (lim-fo-gran-u-LO-ma ve-nar-E-um)

This is a rare disease in the USA, most frequently manifested in heterosexual men as unilateral tender inguinal nodes and in women and homosexual men with proctocolitis, or inflammatory involvement or perirectal or perianal fistulas or strictures

Organism: Invasive strains L1, L2, or L3 of Chlamydia trachomatis

Diagnosis: Serological and exclusion of other ulcerative lesions or those with lymphadenopathy.

Treatment: Treatment cures infection and prevents ongoing tissue damage, although tissue reaction can result in scarring. Buboes may require aspiration through intact skin or incision and drainage to prevent the formation of inguinal/femoral ulcerations.

- ***LGV, Recommended Regimen***
  Doxycycline............................100 mg orally twice a day for 21 days OR
- ***Alternative Regimen***
  Erythromycin base..................500 mg orally four times a day for 21 days

SYPHILIS   (SIF–i–lis)

Organism: *Treponema pallidum* (tre-po-NE-ma PAL-e-dum)
Diagnosis: See most recent CDC Guidelines or ***Contraceptive Technology***
Treatment:
- Parenteral penicillin G is preferred drug for Rx of all stages of syphilis. The preparation(s) used (i.e., benzathine, aqueous procaine, or aqueous crystalline), the dosage, and the length of Rx depend on the stage and clinical manifestations of disease
- Parenteral penicillin G is the only therapy with documented efficacy for neurosyphilis or for syphilis during pregnancy. Patients who report a penicillin allergy, including pregnant women with syphilis in any stage and patients with neurosyphilis, should be desensitized and treated with penicillin
- The Jarisch-Herxheimer reaction is an acute febrile reaction often accompanied by headache, myalgia, and other symptoms that might occur within the first 24 hours after any therapy for syphilis; patients should be advised of this possible adverse reaction

PRIMARY, SECONDARY AND EARLY LATENT SYPHILIS

- ***Recommended Regimen for Adults***
  Benzathine penicillin G....... 2.4 million units IM in a single dose

---

Management Considerations: All patients who have syphilis should be tested for HIV infection. In areas in which the prevalence of HIV is high, patients who have primary syphilis should be retested for HIV after 3 months if the first HIV test result was negative
Follow-up: Serologic test titers may decline more slowly for patients who previously had syphilis. Patients should be reexamined clinically and serologically at both 6 months and 12 months; also see complete *2002 CDC Guidelines* for more detail
Management of Sex Partners: *Sexual transmission of* T. pallidum *has occurred only when mucocutaneous syphilitic lesions are present;* such manifestations are uncommon after the first year of infection. However, persons exposed sexually to a patient who has syphilis in any stage should be evaluated clinically and, according to CDC, serologically
Special Considerations
- *Penicillin Allergy:* Nonpregnant penicillin-allergic patients who have primary or secondary syphilis should be treated with one of the following regimens. Close follow-up of such patients is essential. Limited clinical studies suggest that ceftriaxone may be effective for early syphilis. The optional dose and duration of therapy have not been defined, however, some specialists recommend 1 gm daily IM or IV for 8-10 days

---

- ***Recommended Regimens***
  Doxycycline.............................100 mg orally twice a day for 2 weeks, OR
  Tetracycline.............................500 mg orally four times a day for 2 weeks
- Pregnant patients who are allergic to penicillin should be desensitized, if necessary, and treated with penicillin.

157

See most recent CDC Guidelines or *Contraceptive Technology*
TERTIARY SYPHILIS:
See most recent CDC Guidelines or *Contraceptive Technology*

DISEASES CHARACTERIZED BY URETHRITIS AND CERVICITIS

Management of Patients Who Have Nongonococcal Urethritis

Diagnosis: Testing for chlamydia is strongly recommended because of the increased utility and availability of highly sensitive and specific testing methods and because a specific diagnosis might improve compliance and partner notification

Treatment:

• *Nongonococcal Urethritis, Recommended Regimens*
Azithromycin...........................1 g orally in a single dose, OR
Doxycycline............................100 mg orally twice a day for 7 days

• *Nongonococcal Urethritis, Alternative Regimens*
Erythromycin base.....................500 mg orally four times a day for 7 days, OR
Erythromycin ethylsuccinate....800 mg orally four times a day for 7 days, OR
Ofloxacin.................................300 mg twice a day for 7 days, OR
Levofloxacin............................500 mg orally once daily for 7 days

---

Follow-up: If symptoms persist, patients should be instructed to return for reevaluation and to abstain from sexual intercourse even if they have completed the prescribed therapy

Partner Referral: Patients should refer all sex partners within the preceding 60 days for evaluation and treatment

---

• *Recurrent/Persistent Urethritis, Recommended Treatment*
Metronidazole...........................2 g orally in a single dose, PLUS
Erythromycin base.....................500 mg orally four times a day for 7 days, OR
Erythromycin ethylsuccinate....800 mg orally four times a day for 7 days

---

CHLAMYDIAL INFECTION IN ADOLESCENTS AND ADULTS

Several important sequelae can result from *Chlamydia trachomatis* (kla-MID-e-a tra-KO-ma-tis) infection in women; the most serious of these include PID, ectopic pregnancy, and infertility. Some women who have apparently uncomplicated cervical infection already have subclinical upper reproductive tract infection. Chlamydial infection is much more common in women under age 25 than in older women. Asymptomatic older women need not be screened, but sexually-active young women should be.

Diagnosis: See complete *2002 CDC Guidelines* or *Contraceptive Technology*

Treatment:

• Treatment of infected patients prevents transmission to sex partners and, for infected pregnant women, might prevent transmission to infants during birth
• Treatment of sex partners helps to prevent reinfection of the index patient and infection of other partners
• Coinfection with *C. trachomatis* often occurs among patients who have gonococcal infection; therefore, presumptive treatment of such patients for chlamydia is appropriate (see GONOCOCCAL INFECTION, Dual Therapy for Gonococcal and Chlamydial Infection, p 159)
• The following recommended treatment regimens and the alternative regimens cure infection and usually relieve symptoms:

- *Chlamydia Infection, Recommended Regimens*

Azithromycin..........................1 g orally in a single dose, OR (equally effective)
Doxycycline............................100 mg orally twice a day for 7 days

- *Chlamydia Infection, Alternative Regimens*

Erythromycin base...................500 mg orally four times a day for 7 days, OR
Erythromycin ethylsuccinate...800 mg orally four times a day for 7 days, OR
Ofloxacin................................300 mg orally twice a day for 7 days, OR
Levofloxacin...........................500 mg orally for 7 days

Follow-up: Patients do not need to be retested for chlamydia after completing treatment with doxycycline or azithromycin unless symptoms persist or reinfection is suspected because these therapies are highly efficacious. Consider rescreening for chlamydia infection 3-4 months after treatment due to high prevalence of reinfection, especially for adolescents

Management of Sex Partners: Patients should be instructed to refer their sex partners for evaluation, testing, and treatment, if they had sexual contact with the patient during the 60 days preceding onset of symptoms in the patient or diagnosis of chlamydia

Special Considerations:
- *Pregnancy:*
  - Doxycycline and ofloxacin are contraindicated for pregnant women
  - Azithromycin may be safe/effective though the safety and efficacy of azithromycin use in pregnant and lactating women have not been completely established
  - Repeat testing, preferably by culture, 3 weeks after completion of therapy with the following regimens is recommended because a) none of these regimens is highly efficacious and b) frequent side effects of erythromycin may discourage patient compliance

- *Recommended Regimens for Pregnant Women*

Erythromycin base...................500 mg orally four times a day for 7 days. OR
Amoxicillin.............................500 mg orally three times a day for 7 days.

- *Alternative Regimens for Pregnant Women*

Erythromycin base.....................250 mg orally four times a day for 14 days. OR
Erythromycin ethylsuccinate.....800 mg orally four times a day for 7 days, OR
Erythromycin ethylsuccinate.....400 mg orally four times a day for 14 days, OR
Azithromycin...........................1 g orally in a single dose.

NOTE: Erythromycin estolate is contraindicated during pregnancy because of drug-related hepatotoxicity. Preliminary data indicate that azithromycin may be safe and effective

GONOCOCCAL INFECTION

DUAL THERAPY FOR GONOCOCCAL AND CHLAMYDIAL INFECTIONS

Patients infected with *N. gonorrhoeae* often are coinfected with *C. trachomatis*; this finding led to the recommendation that patients treated for gonococcal infection also be treated routinely with a regimen effective against uncomplicated genital *C. trachomatis* infection

Uncomplicated Gonococcal Infections of the Cervix, Urethra, and Rectum
- *Recommended Regimens*

Cefixime..................................   400 mg orally in a single dose OR
Ceftriaxone.............................125 mg IM in a single dose, OR
Ciprofloxacin..........................500 mg orally in a single dose, OR
Ofloxacin................................400 mg orally in a single dose, OR
Levofloxacin........................... 250 mg orally in a single dose, <u>AND</u>
Azithromycin...........................1 g orally in a single dose, OR
Doxycycline............................100 mg orally twice a day for 7 days

Uncomplicated Gonococcal Infections of the Cervix, Urethra, and Rectum
• Alternative Regimens
Spectinomycin....................2 g IM in a single dose. Spectinomycin is effective, but it is expensive and must be injected. It is useful for treatment of patients who cannot tolerate cephalosporins and quinolones

Single-dose cephalosporin....regimens other than cefritaxone 125 mg IM and cefixime 400 mg include a) ceftizoxime 500 mg IM, b) cefotaxime 500 mg IM, and c) cefoxitin 2 g IM with probenecid 1 g orally

Single-dose quinolone............regimens include gatifloxacin 400 mg orally, lomefloxacin 400 mg orally, and norfloxacin 800 mg orally. None of the regimens appears to offer any advantage over ciprofloxacin or ofloxacin

- Many other antimicrobials are active against *N. gonorrhoeae*
- Azithromycin 2 g orally is effective against uncomplicated gonococcal infection, but it is expensive and causes gastrointestinal distress too often to be recommended for treatment of gonorrhea
- An oral dose of 1 g azithromycin is insufficiently effective and not recommended
- Quinolones (Ciprofloxin, Ofloxacin, Levofloxin) should not be used for infections acquired in Asia or the Pacific, including Hawaii

Uncomplicated Gonococcal Infection of the Pharynx
- Gonococcal infections of the pharynx are more difficult to eradicate than infections at urogenital and anorectal sites
- Few antigonococcal regimens can reliably cure such infections >90% of the time
- Although chlamydial coinfection of the pharynx is unusual, coinfection at genital sites sometimes occurs. Therefore, treatment for both gonorrhea and chlamydia is suggested

• Recommended Regimen
Ceftriaxone............................125 mg IM in a single dose, OR

Ciprofloxacin.........................500 mg orally in a single dose, PLUS

Azithromycin.........................1 g orally in a single dose, OR

Doxycycline...........................100 mg orally twice a day for 7 days

Management of Sex Partners: All sex partners of patients who have *N. gonorrhea* infection should be evaluated and treated for *N. gonorrhea* and *C. trachomatis* infections if their last sexual contact with the patient was within 60 days before onset of symptoms or diagnosis

Special Considerations:
- Pregnant women should not be treated with quinolones or tetracyclines
- Pregnant women infected with *N. gonorrhoeae* should be treated with a recommended or alternate cephalosporin
- Women who cannot tolerate a cephalosporin should be administered a single 2-g dose of spectinomycin IM
- Either erythromycin or amoxicillin is recommended for treatment of presumptive or diagnosed *C. trachomatis* infection during pregnancy (see CHLAMYDIAL INFECTION, p. 158)

DISEASES CHARACTERIZED BY VAGINAL DISCHARGE

Management of Patients Who Have Vaginal Infections:

- Vaginitis is usually characterized by a vaginal discharge or vulvar itching and irritation; a vaginal odor may be present
- The three diseases most frequently associated with vaginal discharge are trichomoniasis (caused by *T. vaginalis*), BV (caused by a replacement of the normal vaginal flora by an overgrowth of anaerobic microorganisms and *Gardnerella vaginalis*), and candidiasis (usually caused by *Candida albicans*)
- Mucopurulent cervicitis caused by *C. trachomatis* or *N. gonorrhoeae* can sometimes cause vaginal discharge
- Vaginitis is diagnosed by pH and microscopic examination of fresh samples of the discharge
- The pH of the vaginal secretions can be determined by narrow-range pH paper for the elevated pH typical of BV or trichomoniasis (i.e., pH of >4.5)
- One way to examine the discharge is to dilute a sample in one to two drops of 0.9% normal saline solution on one slide and 10% potassium hydroxide (KOH) solution on a second slide. Always prepare saline slide first
- An amine odor detected immediately after applying KOH suggests BV
- A cover slip is placed on each slide, which is then examined under a microscope at low and high-dry power. The motile *T. vaginalis* or the clue cells of BV usually are identified easily in the saline specimen
- The yeast or pseudohyphae of *Candida* species are more easily identified in the KOH specimen
- The presence of objective signs of vulvar inflammation in the absence of vaginal pathogens, along with a minimal amount of discharge, suggests the possibility of mechanical, chemical, allergic, or other noninfectious irritation of the vulva
- Culture for *T. vaginalis* is more sensitive than microscopic examination
- Laboratory testing fails to identify the cause of vaginitis among a minority of women

BACTERIAL VAGINOSIS (BV)

- BV is a clinical syndrome resulting from replacement of the normal H_2O_2 producing *Lactobacillus* sp. in the vagina with high concentrations of anaerobic bacteria (e.g., *Prevotella* sp. and *Mobiluncus* sp.), *G. vaginalis*, and *Mycoplasma hominis*
- BV is the most prevalent cause of vaginal discharge or malodor
- Half of women whose illnesses meet the clinical criteria for BV are asymptomatic
- Treatment of male sex partner has not been beneficial in preventing recurrence

Diagnostic Considerations: BV can be diagnosed by the use of clinical criteria meeting three of the following symptoms or signs:

    a. A homogeneous, white, noninflammatory discharge that smoothly coats the vaginal walls

    b. The presence of clue cells on microscopic examination

    c. A pH of vaginal fluid >4.5

    d. A fishy odor of vaginal discharge before or after addition of 10% KOH (i.e., the whiff test)

Treatment: The principal goal of therapy is to relieve vaginal symptoms and signs of infection. All women with symptoms require treatment, regardless of pregnancy status

---

- **BV, Recommended Regimens for Nonpregnant Women**

Metronidazole..................500 mg orally twice a day for 7 days, OR
Clindamycin cream............2%, one full applicator (5 g) intravaginally at bedtime for 7 days OR
Metronidazole gel............0.75%, one full applicator (5 g) intravaginally, once daily for 5 days OR

- Patients should be advised to avoid consuming alcohol during treatment with metronidazole and for 24 hours thereafter. Clindamycin cream is oil-based and might weaken latex condoms and diaphragms

---

- **BV, Alternative Regimens**

Metronidazole........................2 g orally in a single dose, OR

Clindamycin..........................300 mg orally bid x 7 days OR

Clindamycin ovules................100 mg intravaginally qhs x 3 days

---

Recommended metronidazole regimens are equally efficacious. The vaginal clindamycin cream appears to be less efficacious than the metronidazole regimens

- Metronidazole 2 g single-dose therapy is an alternative regimen because of its lower efficacy for BV
- FDA has approved both metronidazole 750-mg extended release tablets once daily for 7 days and metronidazole gel 0.75% once daily intravaginally for 5 days for treatment of BV. However, data concerning clinical equivalency of these regimens with other regimens have not been published. Some health-care providers remain concerned about the possible teratogenicity of metronidazole, which has been suggested by animal experiments; however, a recent meta-analysis does not indicate teratogenicity in humans

Follow-up: Follow-up visits are unnecessary if symptoms resolve. Recurrence is not unusual

- Because treatment of BV in high-risk pregnant women who are asymptomatic might prevent adverse pregnancy outcomes, a follow-up evaluation, at 1 month after completion of treatment, should be considered

Management of Sex Partners: Routine treatment of sex partners is not recommended

Special Considerations:

- *Allergy or Intolerance to the Recommended Therapy:*
  - Clindamycin cream is preferred in case of allergy or intolerance to metronidazole. Metronidazole gel can be considered for patients who do not tolerate systemic metronidazole, but patients allergic to oral metronidazole should not be administered metronidazole vaginally
- *Pregnancy:*
  - BV has been associated with adverse pregnancy outcomes (i.e., premature rupture of the membranes, preterm labor, and preterm birth)
  - Organisms found in increased concentration in BV also are frequently present in postpartum or post-cesarean endometritis
  - Treat all symptomatic pregnant women when diagnosed
  - Treatment of BV in high-risk pregnant women (i.e., those who have previously delivered a premature infant) who are asymptomatic might reduce preterm delivery. However, the optimal treatment regimens have not been established. Some specialists screen and treat those with BV at first prenatal visit
  - The recommended regimen is metronidazole 250 mg orally three times a day for 7 days
  - The alternative regimens are a) metronidazole 2 g orally in a single dose or b) clindamycin 300 mg orally twice a day for 7 days
  - Low-risk pregnant women (i.e., those who previously have not had a premature delivery) who have symptomatic BV should be treated to relieve symptoms. Recommended regimen is metronidazole 250 mg orally three times a day for 7 days
  - Lower doses of medication are recommended for pregnant women to minimize exposure to the fetus. Data are limited concerning the use of metronidazole vaginal gel during pregnancy. Use of clindamycin vaginal cream during pregnancy is not recommended because three randomized trials indicated an increase in the number of preterm deliveries among pregnant women who were treated with this medication

Other: The bacterial flora that characterize BV have been recovered from the endometria and salpinges of women who have PID

TRICHOMONIASIS

Diagnosis:
- Trichomoniasis is caused by the protozoan *T. vaginalis,* easily identified on a wet smear
  Most men who are infected do not have symptoms of infection, although a minority of
  men have nongonococcal urethritis
- Many women do have symptoms of infection, characteristically a diffuse, malodorous,
  yellow-green discharge with vulvar irritation; many women have fewer symptoms
- Vaginal trichomoniasis might be associated with adverse pregnancy outcomes,
  particularly premature rupture of the membranes and preterm delivery

Treatment:
- **Trichomoniasis, Recommended Regimen**
  Metronidazole........................2 g orally in a single dose

- **Trichomoniasis, Alternative Regimen**
  Metronidazole........................500 mg twice a day for 7 days

- Metronidazole is the only oral medication available in the United States
- In randomized clinical trials, the recommended metronidazole regimens have resulted
  in cure rates of approximately 90% - 95%; ensuring treatment of sex partners might
  increase the cure rate. Treatment of patients and sex partners results in relief of
  microbiologic cure, and reduction of transmission
- Discourage use of Metronidazole gel

Follow-up:
- Unnecessary for men and women who become asymptomatic after treatment or who are
  initially asymptomatic
- Infections with strains of *T. vaginalis* that have diminished susceptibility to metronidazole can occur; however, most of these organisms respond to higher doses of metronidazole
- If treatment failure occurs with either regimen, the patient should be retreated with
  metronidazole 500 mg twice a day for 7 days
- If treatment failure occurs repeatedly, the patient should be treated with a single, 2g
  dose of metronidazole once a day for 3-5 days

Management of Sex Partners: Routine Rx recommended avoid intercourse until Rx is
complete and both partners are assymptomatic

Special Considerations:
- *Allergy, Intolerance, or Adverse Reactions:* Effective alternatives to therapy with
  metronidazole are not available. Patients who are allergic to metronidazole can be
  managed by desensitization
- *Pregnancy:* Patients may be treated with 2 g of metronidazole in a single dose
- *HIV Infection:* Patients who have trichomoniasis and also are infected with HIV should
  receive the same treatment regimen as those who are HIV negative

VULVOVAGINAL CANDIDIASIS (VVC)
- Vulvovaginal yeast infections are caused by *C. albicans* or, occasionally, by other
  Candida sps., *Torulopsis* sp., or other yeasts
- An estimated 75% of women will have at least one episode of VVC
- A small percentage of women (i.e., probably <5%) experience recurrent VVC
- Typical symptoms of VVC include pruritus and vaginal discharge
- Other symptoms may include vaginal soreness, vulvar burning, dyspareunia, and external
  dysuria
- None of these symptoms is specific for VVC

Diagnostic Considerations:

- A diagnosis of *Candida* vaginitis is suggested clinically by pruritus and erythema in the vulvo-vaginal area; a white discharge may occur, as may vulvar edema
- The diagnosis can be made in a woman who has signs and symptoms of vaginitis, and when either a) a wet preparation or Gram stain of vaginal discharge demonstrates yeasts or pseudohyphae or b) a culture or other test yields a positive result for a yeast species
- *Candida* vaginitis is associated with a normal vaginal pH (<4.5)
- Use of 10% KOH in wet preparations improves the visualization of yeast and mycelia by disrupting cellular material that might obscure the yeast or pseudohyphae
- Identifying *Candida* by culture in the absence of symptoms should not lead to treatment because 10%-20% of women usually harbor *Candida* sp. and other yeasts in the vagina. VVC can occur concomitantly with STIs or frequently following antibacterial vaginal or systemic therapy

Treatment: Topical formulations effectively treat VVC. The topically applied azole drugs are more effective than nystatin. Treatment with azoles results in relief of symptoms and negative cultures among 80%-90% of patients who complete therapy

---

- **VVC, Recommended Regimens**
- **Intravaginal agents:**

Butoconazole*	2% cream 5 g intravaginally for 3 days, **OR**
Butoconazole*	2% cream 5g (butoconazole 1-sustained release), single vaginal application
Clotrimazole*	1% cream 5 g intravaginally for 7-14 days, **OR**
Clotrimazole*	100-mg vaginal tablet for 7 days, **OR**
Clotrimazole*	100-mg vaginal tablet, two tablets for 3 days, **OR**
Clotrimazole*	500-mg vaginal tablet, one tablet in a single application, **OR**
Miconazole*	2% cream 5 g intravaginally for 7 days, **OR**
Miconazole*	200-mg vaginal suppository, one suppository for 3 days, **OR**
Miconazole*	100-mg vaginal suppository, one suppository for 7 days, **OR**
Nystatin	100,000-u vaginal tablet, one tablet for 14 days, **OR**
Tioconazole*	6.5% ointment 5 g intravaginally in a single application, **OR**
Terconazole*	0.4% cream 5 g intravaginally for 7 days, **OR**
Terconazole*	0.8% cream 5 g intravaginally for 3 days, **OR**
Terconazole*	80-mg vaginal suppository, one suppository for 3 days, **OR**

- **Oral agent:**

Fluconazole	150-mg oral tablet, one tablet in single dose.

---

*These creams and suppositories are oil-based and may weaken latex condoms and diaphragms

- **VVC, Alternative Regimens**
- The ease of administering oral agents is an advantage over topical therapies
- However, the potential for toxicity associated with using a systemic drug, particularly ketoconazole, must be considered

Follow-up: Patients should be instructed to return for follow-up visits only if symptoms persist or recur

Management of Sex Partners: None; VVC usually is not acquired through sexual intercourse

Special Considerations:
- *Pregnancy:* VVC often occurs during pregnancy. Only topical azole therapies should be used to treat pregnant women. Of those treatments that have been investigated for use during pregnancy, the most effective are butoconazole, clotrimazole, miconazole, and terconazole. Many experts recommend 7 days of therapy during pregnancy
- *HIV Infection:* Studies are in progress to confirm an alleged increase in incidence of VVC in HIV-infected women

PELVIC INFLAMMATORY DISEASE (PID) (see Table 13.1, page 39)

- PID comprises a spectrum of inflammatory disorders of the upper female genital tract, including any combination of endometritis, salpingitis, tuboovarian abscess, and pelvic peritonitis
- Sexually transmitted organisms, especially *N. gonorrhoeae* and *C. trachomatis*, are implicated in most cases; however, microorganisms that can be part of the vaginal flora (e.g., anaerobes, *G. vaginalis*, *H. influenzae*, enteric gram negative rods, and *Streptococcus agalactiae*) also can cause PID
- In addition, CMV, *M. hominis* and *U. urealyticum* may also be etiologic agents

Diagnostic Considerations: See complete *2002 CDC Guidelines (www.cdc.gov)*. Empiric treatment should be initiated in sexually active young women and others at risk for STIs if all the following **minimum criteria** are present and no other cause(s) for the illness can be identified:
- Uterine/adenexal tenderness or
- Cervical motion tenderness

Treatment: Must provide empiric, broad-spectrum coverage of likely pathogens
Antimicrobial coverage should include *N. gonorrhea*, *C. trachomatis*, anaerobes, gram-negative facultative bacteria, and streptococci
- *Criteria for **HOSPITALIZATION** based on observational data and theoretical concerns:*
  - Surgical emergencies such as appendicitis cannot be excluded
  - Patient is pregnant
  - Patient does not respond clinically to oral antimicrobial therapy
  - Patient is unable to follow or tolerate an outpatient oral regimen
  - Patient has severe illness, nausea and vomiting, or high fever
  - Patient has a tuboovarian abscess; or

Most clinicians favor at least 24 hours of direct inpatient observation for patients who have tuboovarian abscesses. After that, parenteral therapy should have reduced the risk of abcess progression or rupture

---

- *PID, Parenteral Regimen A*

Cefotetan.................................2 g IV every 12 hours, **OR**
Cefoxitin.................................2 g IV every 6 hours, **PLUS**
Doxycycline............................100 mg IV or orally every 12 hours

- Because of pain associated with infusion, doxycycline should be administered orally when possible, even when the patient is hospitalized
- Both oral and IV administration of doxycycline provide similar bioavailability
- When tuboovarian abscess is present, many health-care providers use clindamycin or metronidazole with doxycycline for continued therapy rather than doxycycline alone, because it provides more effective anaerobic coverage

- **PID, Parenteral Regimen B**

Clindamycin	900 mg IV every 8 hours, **PLUS**
Gentamicin	loading dose IV or IM (2 mg/kg of body weight) followed by a maintenance dose (1.5 mg/kg) every 8 hours. Single daily dosing may be substituted.

- Although use of a single daily dose of gentamicin has not been evaluated for the treatment of PID, it is efficacious in analogous situations
- Parenteral therapy may be discontinued 24 hours after a patient improves clinically, and continuing oral therapy should consist of doxycycline 100 mg orally twice a day or clindamycin 450 mg orally four times a day to complete a total of 14 days of therapy
- When tuboovarian abscess is present, many healthcare providers use clindamycin for continued anaerobic coverage rather than doxycycline because clindamycin provides more effective anaerobic coverage

- **PID, Alternative Parenteral Regimens:** Limited data support the use of other parenteral regimens, but the following three regimens have been investigated in at least one clinical trial, and they have broad-spectrum coverage.

Ofloxacin	400 mg IV every 12 hours, OR Levofloxacin 500 mg IV once daily with or without metronidazole 500 mg IV every 8 hours **OR**
Ampicillin/Sulbactam	3 g IV every 6 hours, PLUS doxycycline 100 mg IV / orally every 12 hours **OR**

Oral Treatment: The following regimens provide coverage against the frequent etiologic agents of PID, but evidence from clinical trials supporting their use is limited. Patients who do not respond to oral therapy within 72 hours should be reevaluated to confirm the diagnosis and administered parenteral therapy on either an outpatient or inpatient basis.

- **PID, Oral Regimen A**

Ofloxacin	400 mg orally twice a day for 14 days, **OR**
Levofloxacin	500 mg daily for 14 days, WITH or WITHOUT
Metronidazole	500 mg orally twice a day for 14 days.

- **PID, Oral Regimen B**

Ceftriaxone	250 mg IM once, **OR**
Cefoxitin	2 g IM plus probenecid, 1 g orally in a single dose concurrently once, **OR**

Other parenteral third-generation cephalosporin (e.g.,ceftizoxime or cefotaxime), **PLUS**

Doxycycline	100 mg orally twice a day for 14 days with or without metronidazole 500 mg orally twice daily for 14 days.

Follow-up:
- Patients receiving oral or parenteral Rx should demonstrate substantial clinical improvement (i.e., defervescence; reduction in direct or rebound abdominal tenderness; and reduction in uterine, adnexal, and Cx motion tenderness) within 3 days after initiation of Rx
- Patients who do not improve within 3 days usually require additional diagnostic tests, surgical intervention, or both
- If the health-care provider prescribes outpatient oral or parenteral therapy, a follow-up examination should be performed within 72 hours

Special Considerations:
- *Pregnancy:* Pregnant women who have suspected PID should be hospitalized and treated with parenteral antibiotics.

Genital Warts: An effective vaccine is on the way! ←

- More than 30 types of HPV can infect the genital tract. Most HPV infections are asymptomatic, subclinical, or unrecognized. Visible genital warts usually are caused by HPV types 6 or 11. Other HPV types in the anogenital region (i.e., types 16, 18, 31, 33, and 35) have been strongly associated with cervical dysplasia
- No data support the use of type-specific HPV nucleic acid tests in the routine diagnosis or management of visible genital warts
- HPV types 6 and 11 also can cause warts on the uterine cervix and in the vagina, urethra, and anus; these warts are sometimes symptomatic
- HPV types 6 and 11 are associated rarely with invasive squamous cell carcinoma of the external genitalia
- HPV types 16, 18, 31, 33, and 35 are found occasionally in visible genital warts and have been associated with external genital (i.e., vulvar, penile, and anal) squamous intraepithelial neoplasia (i.e., squamous cell carcinoma in situ, bowenoid papulosis, erythroplasia of Queyrat, or Bowen's disease of the genitalia). These HPV types have been associated with vaginal, anal, and cervical intraepithelial dysplasia and squamous cell carcinoma. Patients who have visible genital warts can be infected simultaneously with multiple HPV types

Treatment:

- The primary goal of treating visible genital warts is the removal of symptomatic warts
- Treatment can induce wart-free periods in most patients. Genital warts often are asymptomatic
- **No evidence indicates that currently available treatments eradicate or affect the natural history of HPV infection.** The removal of warts may or may not decrease infectivity
- If left untreated, visible genital warts may resolve on their own, remain unchanged, or increase in size or number. No evidence indicates that treatment of visible warts affects the development of cervical cancer

Regimens:

- Treatment of genital warts should be guided by the patient's preference, the available resources, and the experience of the health-care provider.
- None of the available treatments is superior to other treatments, and no single treatment is ideal for all circumstances. The treatment modality should be changed if a patient has not improved substantially after three provider-administered treatments or if warts have not completely cleared after six treatments
- Providers should be knowledgeable about, and have available, at least one patient-applied and one provider-administered treatment

---

- ***External Genital Warts, Recommended Treatments:***
- *Patient-Applied*

Podofilox..............................0.5% solution or gel.

- Patients may apply podofilox solution with a cotton swab, or podofilox gel with a finger, to visible genital warts twice a day for 3 days, followed by 4 days of no therapy
- This cycle may be repeated as necessary for a total of four cycles
- The total wart area treated should not exceed 10 cm², and a total volume of podofilox should not exceed 0.5 mL per day
- If possible, the health-care provider should apply the initial treatment to demonstrate the proper application technique and identify which warts should be treated. The safety

of podofilox during pregnancy has not been established. **OR**

Imiquimod..............................5% cream.
- Patients should apply imiquimod cream with a finger at bedtime, three times a week for as long as 16 weeks
- The treatment area should be washed with mild soap and water 6-10 hours after the application
- Many patients may be clear of warts by 8-10 weeks or sooner
- The safety of imiquimod during pregnancy has not been established

- *Provider-Administered:*
  Cryotherapy with liquid nitrogen or cryoprobe. Repeat applications every 1 to 2 weeks **OR**
  Trichloroacetic acid (TCA) or BCA 80%-90%. May place petroleum jelly around wart to reduce spread of medication to normal mucosa. Apply a small amount only to warts and allow to dry, at which time a white "frosting" develops; powder with talc or $NaHCO_3$ to remove unreacted acid if an excess amount is applied. Repeat weekly if necessary. **OR**
  Podophyllin resin....................10%-25% in tincture of benzoin
- A small amount should be applied to each wart and allowed to air dry
- To avoid the possibility of complications associated with systemic absorption and toxicity, some experts recommend that application be limited to <0.5 mL of podophyllin or <10 cm^2 of warts per session
- Some experts suggest that the preparation should be thoroughly washed off 1-4 hours after application to reduce local irritation. Repeat weekly if necessary
- *The safety of podophyllin during pregnancy has not been established*
- *Surgical removal* by tangential scissor excision, tangential shave excision, curettage, or electrosurgery

- **External Genital Warts, Alternative Treatments (Provider administered)**
  Intra-lesional interferon **OR**
  Laser surgery

- **Cervical Warts**
  For women who have exophytic cervical warts, high-grade squamous intraepithelial lesions (SIL) must be excluded before treatment is begun. Management of exophytic cervical warts should include consultation with an expert

- **Vaginal Warts, Recommended Treatment**
  Cryotherapy with liquid nitrogen. The use of a cryoprobe in the vagina is not recommended because of the risk for vaginal perforation and fistula formation. **OR**
  TCA or BCA 80%-90% applied only to warts. Repeat weekly if necessary.

- **Urethral Meatus Warts, Recommended Treatment**
  Cryotherapy with liquid nitrogen **OR**
  Podophyllin 10%-25% in tincture of benzoin. The treatment area must be dry before contact with normal mucosa. Podophyllin must be applied weekly if necessary. *The safety of podophyllin during pregnancy has not been established.*

• **Anal Warts, Recommended Treatment**
Cryotherapy with liquid nitrogen **OR**

TCA or BCA 80%-90% applied to warts. Apply a small amount only to warts and allow to dry, at which time a white "frosting" develops; powder with talc or sodium bicarbonate (i.e., baking soda) to remove unreacted acid if an excess amount is applied. Repeat weekly if necessary. May place petroleum jelly around wart to reduce spread of medication to normal mucosa **OR**
Surgical removal

• Management of warts on rectal mucosa should be referred to an expert

Follow-up: After visible genital warts have cleared, a follow-up is not mandatory
Management of Sex Partners: None. Examination of sex partners is not necessary for the management of genital warts because the role of reinfection is probably minimal and, in the absence of curative therapy, treatment to reduce transmission is not realistic
Special Considerations:

• *Pregnancy:* Imiquimod, podophyllin, and podofilox should not be used during pregnancy. Because genital warts can proliferate and become friable during pregnancy, many experts advocate their removal during pregnancy. HPV types 6 and 11 can cause laryngeal papillomatosis in infants and children. Vaginal delivery not contraindicated unless lesion size obstructive in labor (rare). The route of transmission (i.e., transplacental, perinatal, or postnatal) is not completely understood

VACCINE-PREVENTABLE STIs

One of the most effective means of preventing the transmission of STIs is preexposure immunization. Currently licensed vaccines for the prevention of STIs include those for hepatitis A and hepatitis B. Clinical development and trials are underway for vaccines against a number of other STIs, including HIV and HSV. As more vaccines become available, immunization possibly will become one of the most widespread methods used to prevent STIs

ECTOPARASITIC INFECTIONS

PEDICULOSIS PUBIS

Patients who have pediculosis pubis (i.e., pubic lice) usually seek medical attention because of pruritus. Such patients also usually notice lice or nits on their pubic hair

Treatment:
• **Pediculosis Pubis, Recommended Regimens**
Permethrin...........................1% creme rinse applied to affected areas and washed off after 10 minutes **OR**
Lindane................................1% shampoo applied for 4 minutes to the affected area, and then thoroughly washed off. This regimen is not recommended for pregnant or lactating women or for children aged <2 yrs **OR**
Pyrethrins with piperonyl butoxide applied to the affected area and washed off after 10 minutes.

Other Management Considerations:

• The recommended regimens should not be applied to the eyes. Pediculosis of the eyelashes should be treated by applying occlusive ophthalmic ointment to the eyelid margins twice a day for 10 days
• Bedding and clothing should be decontaminated (either machine-washed and machine-dried using the heat cycle or drycleaned) or removed from body contact for at least 72 hrs
• Fumigation of living areas is not necessary

Follow-up: Patients should be evaluated after 1 week if symptoms persist. Retreatment may be necessary if lice are found or if eggs are observed at the hairskin junction. Patients who do not respond to one of the recommended regimens should be retreated with an alternative regimen

Management of Sex Partners: Sex partners within the last month should be treated

Special Considerations:

- *Pregnancy:* Pregnant and lactating women should be treated with either permethrin or pyrethrins with piperonyl butoxide

SCABIES

- Predominant symptoms is pruritus; sensitization takes several weeks to develop; pruritus might occur within 24 hours after a subsequent reinfestation
- Scabies in adults may be sexually transmitted, although scabies in children usually is not

- *Scabies, Recommended Regimen*

Permethrin cream.................(5%) applied to all areas of the body from the neck down and washed off after 8-14 hours.

- *Scabies, Alternative Regimens*

Lindane.................(1%) 1 oz. of lotion or 30 g of cream applied thinly to all areas of the body from the neck down and thoroughly washed off after 8 hours **OR**

Ivermectin.................200 mg/kg orally, repeated in 2 weeks

- Lindane should not be used immediately after a bath, and it should not be used by a) persons who have extensive dermatitis, b) pregnant or lactating women, and c) children aged <2 years.

Other Management Considerations: Bedding and clothing should be decontaminated (i.e., either machine-washed or machine-dried using the hot cycle or dry-cleaned) or removed from body contact for at least 72 hours. Fumigation of living areas is unnecessary

Follow-up: Pruritus may persist for several weeks. Some experts recommend retreatment after 1 week for patients who are still symptomatic; other experts recommend retreatment only if live mites are observed. Patients who do not respond should be retreated with an alternative regimen

Management of Sex Partners and Household Contacts: Both sexual and close personal or household contacts within the preceding month should be examined and treated

SEXUAL ASSAULT AND STIs: Adults and Adolescents

Evaluation for Sexually Transmitted Infections

- *Initial Examination* - (See inside back cover)
- *Follow-up Examination after Assault*
    - Examination for STIs should be repeated 2 weeks after assault (see inside back cover)
    - Serologic tests for syphilis and HIV infection should be repeated 6, 12, and 24 weeks after the assault if initial test results were negative
- Prophylaxis: Many experts recommend routine preventive therapy after a sexual assault. The prophylactic regimen suggested is on inside back cover
- An empiric antimicrobial regimen for chlamydia, gonorrhea, trichomonas, and BV should be administered (See inside back cover)

Other Management Considerations:

At the initial examination and, if indicated, at follow-up, patients should be counseled about:

- Risk for pregnancy and possible use of emergency contraception
- Symptoms of STIs and the need for immediate examination if symptoms occur
- Abstinence from sexual intercourse until STI prophylactic treatment is completed

Risk for Acquiring HIV Infection:

- Although HIV antibody seroconversion has been reported among persons whose only known risk factor was sexual assault or sexual abuse, the risk for acquiring HIV infection through sexual assault is low and depends on many factors
- These factors may include the type of sexual intercourse (i.e., oral, vaginal, or anal); presence of oral, vaginal or anal trauma; site of exposure to ejaculate; viral load in ejaculate; and presence of an STI

HIV INFECTION

OraQuick, a rapid test (40-60 minutes) was approved by the FDA in November, 2002.
For entire guidelines see www.aidsinfo.nih.gov

Proper management of HIV infection involves a complex array of behavioral, pyschosocial, and medical services. This information should not be a substitute for referral to a health-care provider or facility experienced in caring for HIV-infected patients. Hotlines:

CDC AIDS Treatment Information Service.........1-800-HIV-0440 (1-800-448-0440)
    e-mail to: atis@hivatis.org & www.hivatis.org
CDC AIDS Clinical Trials Information Service....1-800-TRIALS-A (1-800-874-2572)
    e-mailto: actis@actis.org   International....1-301-519-0459
For general information and referrals to local facilities:
CDC National AIDS Hotline................................1-800-342-AIDS (1-800-342-2437)
    Spanish...1-800-344-7432
CDC National AIDS Clearinghouse......................1-800-458-5231
CDC Division of HIV/AIDS Prevention................www.cdc.gov/hiv
Post exposure prophylaxis PEP...........................1-888-HIV-4911

Pregnancy: All pregnant women should be offered HIV testing as early in pregnancy as possible. This recommendation is particularly important because of the available treatments for reducing the likelihood of perinatal transmission and maintaining the health of the woman. HIV-infected women should be informed specifically about the risk for perinatal infection. Current evidence indicates that 15%-25% of infants born to untreated HIV-infected mothers are infected with HIV; the virus also can be transmitted from an infected mother by breastfeeding. Zidovudine (ZDV) reduces the risk for HIV transmission to the infant from approximately 25% to 8% if administered to women during the later stage of pregnancy and during labor and to infants for the first 6 weeks of life. Therefore, **ZDV TREATMENT SHOULD BE OFFERED TO ALL HIV-INFECTED PREGNANT WOMEN**. Most women in the U.S. now receive triple therapy during pregnancy not just ZDV. In the United States, HIV-infected women should be advised not to breast-feed their infants. In other countries, the reduced risk of death from malnutrition, diarrheal disease, or other infections may outweigh the risk of contracting HIV.

Insufficient information is available regarding the safety of ZDV or other antiretroviral drugs during early pregnancy; however, on the basis of the ACTG-076 protocol, ZDV is indicated for the prevention of maternal-fetal HIV transmission as part of a regimen that includes oral ZDV at 14-34 weeks of gestation, intravenous (IV) ZDV during labor, and ZDV syrup to the neonate after birth.

WHO MEDICAL ELIGIBILITY CRITERIA FOR STARTING CONTRACEPTIVE METHODS (2004)

The table on the following pages summarizes the latest World Health Organization (WHO) medical eligibility criteria for starting contraceptives. These criteria are also the basis for the checklists throughout *Managing Contraception*. These criteria are for the most part evidence-based. References are available through the World Health Organization

WHO categories for temporary methods:

WHO 1   **Can use** the method. No restriction on use.

WHO 2   **Can use** the method. Advantages generally outweigh theoretical or proven risks. If method is chosen, more than usual follow-up may be needed.

WHO 3   **Should not use** the method unless clinician makes clinical judgment that the patient can safely use it. **Theoretical or proven risks usually outweigh the advantages** of method. Method of last choice, for which regular monitoring may be needed.

WHO 4   **Should not use** the method. Condition represents an unacceptable health risk if method is used.

Simplified 2-category system for temporary methods

To make clinical judgment, the WHO 4-category classification system can be simplified into a 2-category system.

WHO Category	With Clinical Judgment	With Limited Clinical Judgment
1	Use the method in any circumstances	Use the method
2	Generally use the method	
3	Use of the method not usually recommended unless other, more appropriate methods are not available or acceptable	Do not use the method
4	Method not to be used	

NOTE: In the pages that follow, Category 3 and 4 conditions are shaded to indicate the method should not be provided where clinical judgment is limited.

To download most recent WHO Medical Eligibility Criteria go to: www.whi.mec

WHO MEDICAL ELIGIBILITY CRITERIA FOR STARTING CONTRACEPTIVE METHODS (2004)

To download most recent WHO Medical Eligibility Criteria go to: www.who.mec

CONDITION	Combined OCs	Combined Injectables	Progestin-Only OCs	Depo-Provera NET EN	LNG/ETG Implants	TCu-380A IUD	LNG IUD
PERSONAL CHARACTERISTICS & REPRODUCTIVE HISTORY							
Pregnant	NA	NA	NA	NA	NA	4	4
Age	Menarche to <40=1; ≥40=2	Menarche to <40=1; ≥40=2	Menarche to <18=1; 18-45=1; >45=1	Menarche to <18=2; 18-45=1; >45=2	Menarche to <45=1; >45=1	<20=2; ≥20=1	<20=2; ≥20=1
Parity a) nulliparous*	1	1	1	1	1	2	2
b) parous	1	1	1	1	1	1	1
Breastfeeding < 6 weeks PP	4	4	3	3	3		
≥ 6 weeks to 6 months PP primarily breastfeeding	3	3	1	1	1		
≥ 6 months PP	2	2	1	1	1		
Postpartum < 21 days	3	3	1	1	1		
≥ 21 days	1	1	1	1	1	<48 hrs 3**; 48h-<4 wks 3**; ≥4 wks 1*	<48 hrs 3**; 48h-<4 wks 3**; >4 wks 1*
Puerperal Sepsis						4	4
Post-abortion 1st trimester	1	1	1	1	1	1	1
2nd trimester	1	1	1	1	1	2	2
Immediate post septic AB	1	1	1	1	1	4	4
Past ectopic pregnancy	1	1	2	1	1	1	1

For women older than 45 there are concerns regarding hypo-estrogenic effect of DMPA on bone mass.

There is concern that the neonate may be at risk of exposure to steroid hormones during the first 6 weeks. POCs may be one of the few types of methods available and accessible to breastfeeding women immediately postpartum.

* There are conflicting data regarding whether IUD use is associated with infertility among nulliparous women, although recent well-conducted studies suggest no increased risk

** Breastfeeding or nonbreastfeeding, including post-caesarean section

A2

	COCs	CI	POPs	DMPA	LNG/ETG	TCuIUD	LNGIUD
History of pelvic surgery	1	1	1	1	1	1	1
Smoking: Less than age 35	2	2	1	1	1	1	1
Age ≥ 35 < 15 cigarettes/day	3	2	1	1	1	1	1
Age ≥ 35 ≥ 15 cigarettes/day	4	3	1	1	1	1	1
Obesity > 30 kg/m² BMI	2	2	1	1	1	1	1
CARDIOVASCULAR DISEASE							
Multiple risk factors for CAD (older age, smoking, diabetes, HBP)	3 or 4	3 or 4	2	3	2	1	2
HBP Hx, HBP, BP can't be evaluated	3	3	2	2	2	1	2
HBP adequately controlled	3	3	1	2	1	1	1
BP systolic 140-159 or Diastolic 90-99	3	3	1	2	1	1	1
BP systolic ≥ 160 or Diastolic 100	4	4	2	3	2	1	2
Vascular disease	4	4	2	3	2	1	2
HBP during pregnancy, BP now normal	2	2	1	1	1	1	1
Deep vein thrombosis/pulmonary embolism							
a) History of DVT/PE	4	4	2	2	2	1	2
b) Current DVT/PE	4	4	3	3	3	1	3
c) Family history (first-degree relatives)	2	2	1	1	1	1	1
d) Major surgery with prolonged immobilization	4	4	2	2	2	1	2
e) Major surgery without prolonged immobilization	2	2	1	1	1	1	1
f) Minor surgery without immobilization	1	1	1	1	1	1	1
KNOWN THROMBOGENIC MUTATIONS (e.g. Factor V Leiden, Prothrombin mutation, Protein S, Protein C and Antithrombin deficiencies)	4	4	2	2	2	1	2

When multiple major risk factors exist, risk of CV disease may increase substantially. Some POPs may increase risk of thrombosis although this risk is substantially less than with COCs.

To download most recent WHO Medical Eligibility Criteria go to: www.who.mec.

A3

WHO MEDICAL ELIGIBILITY CRITERIA FOR STARTING CONTRACEPTIVE METHODS (CONTINUED)

To download most recent WHO Medical Eligibility Criteria go to: www.who.mec.

CONDITION	Combined OCs	Combined Injectables	OCs Progestin-Only	Depo-Provera NET EN	LNG/ETG Implants	TCu-380A IUD	LNG IUD	
Superficial venous thrombosis								
a) varicose veins	1	1	1	1	1	1	1	→ Varicose Veins are not risk factors for DVT/PE
b) superficial thrombophlebitis	2	2	2	2	2	1	1	
Current & history of ischemic heart disease	4	4	2/3*	3	2/3	1	2/3	→ There is concern regarding reduced HDL levels among POC users. Some POCs may increase the risk of arterial thrombosis, although this increase is substantially less than with COCs as is associated with hypertensive women only.
Stroke (history of CVA)	4	4	2/3	3	2/3	1	2	
Known hyperlipidemia (screening NOT necessary)	2* or 3*	2 or 3	2	2	2	1	2	
Valvular heart disease uncomplicated	2	2	1	1	1	1	1	
Valvular heart disease complicated	4	4	1	1	1	2	2	
NEUROLOGIC CONDITIONS								
Headaches								
a) non-migraine (mild or severe)	1/2	1/2	1/1	1/1	1/1	1	1/1	
b) migraine < 35, no aura	2/3	2/3	1/2	2/2	2/2	1	2/2	→ New evidence: Among women with migraines, women who also have focal neurologic symptoms have a higher risk of stroke than those without focal neurologic symptoms. In addition, among women with migraines, those who use COCs have a 2 to 4-fold increased risk of stroke compared with women who do not use COCs.
c) migraine ≥ 35, no aura	3/4	3/4	1/2	2/2	2/2	1	2/2	
d) migraine with aura (any age)	4/4	4/4	2/3	2/3	2/3	1	2/3	
Epilepsy	1	1	1	1	1	1	1	
Depressive Disorders	1	1	1	1	1	1	1	
REPRODUCTIVE TRACT INFECTIONS & DISORDERS								
Irregular without heavy bleeding	1	1	2	2	2	1	1/1	
Heavy or prolonged vaginal bleeding (regular or irregular)	1	1	2	2	2	2	1/2	
Unexplained vaginal bleeding. Suspicious for serious underlying condition. Before evaluation	2	2	2	3	3	4/2	4/2	

* Initiation: 2 and Continuation: 3 expressed as 2/3 (I/C)

** If distinction is made between levels of severity of a condition it is expressed as 2 or 3

Condition					
Endometriosis	1	1	1	1	2	1
Benign ovarian tumors (including cysts)	1	1	1	1	1	1
Severe dysmenorrhea	1	1	1	1	2	1
Benign gestational trophoblastic disease	1	1	1	3	3
Malignant gestational trophoblastic disease	1	1	1	4	4
Cervical ectropion	1	1	1	1	1
Cervical intraepithelial neoplasia (CIN)	2	2	2	2	1	2
Cervical cancer (awaiting treatment)	2	2	2	2	4/2	4/2
Undiagnosed breast mass	2	2	2	1	2
Benign breast disease	1	1	1	1	1
Family history of breast cancer	1	1	1	1	1
Breast cancer (current)	4	4	4	4	4
Past breast cancer; No current disease for 5 years	3	3	3	3	3
Endometrial cancer	1	1	1	4/2	4/2
Ovarian cancer	1	1	1	3/2	3/2
Uterine fibroids *without* distortion of uterine cavity	1	1	1	1	1
Uterine fibroids *with* distortion of uterine cavity	1	1	1	4	4

→ Copper IUD may worsen dysmenorrhea associated with endometriosis

→ There is some concern that COCs enhance the progression of CIN to invasive disease, particularly with long-term use

→ Breast cancer is hormonally sensitive, and the prognosis of women with current or recent breast cancer may worsen with COC or POC use

To download most recent WHO Medical Eligibility Criteria go to: www.who.mec.

WHO MEDICAL ELIGIBILITY CRITERIA FOR STARTING CONTRACEPTIVE METHODS (CONTINUED)

To download most recent WHO Medical Eligibility Criteria go to: www.who.mec.

CONDITION	Combined OCS	Combined Injectables	Progestin-Only OCS	Depo-Provera NET EN	Implants LNG/ETG	TCu-380A IUD	LNG IUD	
Past history PID (no current STI risk factors) with subsequent pregnancy	1	1	1	1	1	1/1	1/1	
Past history PID (no current STI risk factors) without subsequent pregnancy	1	1	1	1	1	2/2	2/2	In women at low risk of STIs, IUD insertion poses little risk of PID.
Current PID (or within last 3 months)	1	1	1	1	1	4/2	4/2	Four to insert, number 2 to continue IUD use if PID is treated with appropriate antibiotics
Current purulent cervicitis or chlamydial infection or gonorrhea	1	1	1	1	1	4/2	4/2	
Other STIs (excluding HIV & hepatitis)	1	1	1	1	1	2/2	2/2	
Vaginitis (including trichomonas vaginalis & bacterial vaginosis)	1	1	1	1	1	2	2	
Increased risk of STIs	1	1	1	1	1	2/3/3	2/3/3	
HIV/AIDS								
High risk of HIV	1	1	1	1	1	2/2	2/2	Women at high risk of HIV are also at high risk of other STIs
HIV-positive	1	1	1	1	1	2/2	2/2	
AIDS	1	1	1	1	1	3/2	3/2	
Clinically well on ARV therapy	1	1	1	1	1	2/2	2/2	
ENDOCRINE CONDITIONS								
History gestational diabetes	1	1	1	1	1	1	1	
Non-insulin dependent diabetes (non-vascular disease)	2	2	2	2	2	1	2	
Insulin dependent diabetes (non-vascular disease)	2	2	2	2	2	1	2	There is concern about the possible negative effect of DMPA on lipid metabolism, possibly affecting the progression of nephropathy, retinopathy or other vascular disease
Diabetic nephropathy/retinopathy/neuropathy	3/4	3/4	2	3	2	1	2	
Other vascular disease; diabetes of > 20 years	3/4	3/4	2	3	2	1	2	

CONDITION	Combined OCs	Combined Injectables	Progestin-Only OCs	NET EN Depo-Provera	LNG/ETG Implants	TCu-380A IUD	LNG IUD
Thyroid: simple goiter	1	1	1	1	1	1	1
Hyperthyroid	1	1	1	1	1	1	1
Hypothyroid	1	1	1	1	1	1	1
GASTROINTESTINAL CONDITIONS							
Symptomatic gall bladder disease post cholecystectomy	2	2	2	2	2	1	2
Symptomatic gall bladder disease medically treated	3	2	2	2	2	1	2
Symptomatic gall bladder disease - current	3	2	2	2	2	1	2
Asymptomatic gall bladder disease	2	2	2	2	2	1	2
History of pregnancy-related cholestasis	2	2	1	1	1	1	1
Past COC-related cholestasis	3	2	2	2	2	1	2
Viral hepatitis active	4	3/4*	3	3	3	1	3
Viral hepatitis carrier	1	1	1	1	1	1	1
Cirrhosis: mild compensated	3	2	2	2	2	1	2
Cirrhosis: severe (decompensated)	4	3	3	3	3	3	3
Benign hepatic adenoma	4	3	3	3	3	1	3
Malignant liver tumor (hepatoma)	4	3/4	3	3	3	1	3

*Initiation: 3 and Continuation: 4 expressed as 3/4 (I/C)

COCs may cause small increased risk of gall bladder disease. There is also concern that COCs may worsen existing gallbladder disease

COCs are metabolized by liver and use may adversely affect women whose liver function is already compromised. There is concern about the hormonal load associated with POC use, but it is less than for COCs

A7

WHO MEDICAL ELIGIBILITY CRITERIA FOR STARTING CONTRACEPTIVE METHODS (CONTINU

To download most recent WHO Medical Eligibility Criteria go to: www.who.mec.

CONDITION	Combined OCs	Combined Injectables	Progestin-Only OCs	Depo-Provera NET EN	LNG/ETG implants	TCu-380A IUD	LNG IUD
ANEMIAS							
Thalassemia	1	1	1	1	1	2	1
Sickle cell disease	2	2	1	1	1	2	1
Iron deficiency anemia	1	1	1	1	1	2	1
DRUG INTERACTIONS							
Rifampicin	3	2	3	2	3	1	1
Certain anticonvulsants: Phenytoin, barbiturates carbamazepine, primidone, topiramate, oxycarbazepine	3	2	3	2	3	1	1
Griseofulvin	2	1	2	1	2	1	1
Other antibiotics	1	1	1	1	1	1	1
ANTIRETROVIRAL THERAPY	2	2	2	2	2	2/3	2/3

Although the interaction between commonly used liver enzyme inducers and COCs is not harmful to women, it is likely to reduce the efficacy of COCs. Use of other contraceptives should be encouraged for women who are long-term users of any of these drugs. Whether increasing the hormone dose of COCs is of benefit remains unclear.

HISTORY OF CONTRACEPTION AND POPULATION GROWTH

"We have not inherited the earth from our grandparents, we have borrowed it from our grandchildren."
— Professor John Guillebaud-Attributed to the Ancient Chinese

2005	Subcutaneous Depo-Provera and Implanon approved	
2003	Seasonale, an extended-use pill (0.15 mg LNG, 0.03 mg EE), approved and marketed	
2001	Ortho Evra Patch and NuvaRing approved	1999 - 6 billion
2000	RU486 (mifepristone), Lunelle and Mirena approved by FDA	(10/12/99!!)
1999	World population hits 6 billion (this billion took 12 years)	
1997	FDA approves Emergency Contraceptive Pills	
1994	Plastic (polyurethane) condom for men (Avanti)	
1993	FDA approves polyurethane (plastic) female condom (Reality)	
1992	FDA approves Depo-Provera (DMPA) injections	
1988	Copper T 380-A IUD marketing begins, 5 years after FDA approval	
1987	World population reaches 5 billion (this billion took 12 years)	1987 - 5 billion
1983	FDA approves Copper T 380-A and the Today sponge	
1982	Baulieu describes medical abortion using mifepristone	
1981	First documented case of HIV/AIDS	
1981	Garret Hardin writes "nobody ever dies of overpopulation" after 500,000 die from flooding of an overcrowded East Bengal River delta	
1975	World population reaches 4 billion (this billion took 15 years)	
1974	Al Yuzpe describes emergency contraception using Ovral pills	1975 - 4 billion
1973	FDA approved progestin-only pills (minipills)	
1973	U.S. Supreme Court abortion decision (Roe v Wade & Doe v Bolton)	
1965	U.S. Supreme Court overturns anti-birth control laws in most states (Griswold v. CT)	
1965	U.S. Agency of International Development initiates Population Program	
1960	Food and Drug Administration approves combined oral contraceptives	
1960	World population reaches 3 billion (this billion took 30 years)	
1942	American Birth Control League renamed Planned Parenthood	
1937	AMA ends longstanding opposition to contraception	
1936	German gynecologist Friedrich Wilde describes first cervical cap (fitted from a wax impression)	
1930-31	Knaus (Austria) and Ogino (Japan) develop rhythm method	
1930	World population now 2 billion (this billion took 100 years)	1960 - 3 billion
1930	Pope Pius XI virulently attacks both contraception and abortion	
1927	Novak (Hopkins) describes suction as means of performing an abortion	
1918	N.Y. court approves condoms to prevent disease only	
1916	Margaret Sanger opens first Amercian birth control clinic in Brooklyn, NY	
1914	Margaret Sanger coins word "birth control"	
1912	Sadie Sachs post-abortion death affects Margaret Sanger profoundly	
1909	German surgeon Richard Richter reports success with silkworm-gut shaped into a ring	
1893	First vasectomy by Harrison in London	1930 - 2 billion
1882	First contraceptive clinic established in Amsterdam	
1880	First tubal ligation	
1873	Comstock Act: classifies birth control devices and information as obscene	
1839	Charles Goodyear discovers vulcanization technology; quickly leads to rubber condoms	
1830	World population reaches 1 billion (this billion took 6 million years)	
1798	Thomas Robert Malthus proposes dismal theory that population growth eventually will exceed the ability of the earth to provide food	1800 - 1 billion
Late 1770s	Casanova popularizes condoms for infection control and contraception	
1 AD	World population reaches 250 million, abstinence (particularly postpartum), withdrawal, lactation, stones in camels, lemons for mechanical and spermicidal effect, abortion using molokeeia (same stem used today), homosexuality and polygamy	

1 AD - 250 million

Special thanks to Andrea Tone at Georgia Tech

REFERENCES

Amba J, Chandra A, Mosher V D et al. Fertility, family planning, and women's health: New data from 1995 NSFG. Vital Health Stat 1997; 23:62-63.

American College of Obstetrics and Gynecologists (ACOG). Emergency oral contraception. ACOG Practice Patterns 1996 (Dec. no. 3).

Anderson FD, Hait H, the Seasonale-301 Study Group. A multicenter, randomized study of an extended cycle oral contraceptive. Contraception 2003; 68; 89-96.

Arevalo N, Jennings V, Sinai I. Efficacy of a new method of family planning: the Standard Days Method. Contraception. 2001; 65:333-338.

Artz, L, Demand M, Pulley LV, Posner SF, Macaluso M. Predictors of difficulty inserting the female condom. Contraception 65, 2002:151-157.

Association for Voluntary Surgical Contraception. Postpartum IUD insertion: Clinical and programatic guidelines (monograph) 1994 (AVSC has changed name to Engender Health).

Audet MC, Moreau M, Koltun WD, Waldbaum AS, Shangold G, Fisher AC, Creasy MD. Evaluation of contraceptive efficacy and cycle control of a transdermal contraceptive patch vs. an oral contraceptive: a randomized controlled trial. JAMA. 285;2001:2347-2354.

Backman T, Huhtala S, Luoto R, Tuominen J, Rauramo I, Koskenvuo M. Advance Information Improves User Satisfaction with the Levonorgestrel Intrauterine System. Obstetrics and Gynecology. 99, 2002: 608-13.

Ballagh SA. Sterilization in the office: the concept is now a reality. Contraceptive Technology Reports. February, 2003 supplement to the newsletter, Contraceptive Technology Update.

Barone MA, Nazerali H, Cortez M, et al. A prospective study of time and number of ejaculations to azoospermia after vasectomy by ligation and excision. J Urology 2003; 170:892-896.

Berel V, Hermon C, Kay C, Hannaford P, Darby S, Reeves G. Mortality associated with oral contraceptive use: 25 year follow-up of cohort of 46,000 women from Royal College of General Practitioners' oral contraceptive study; Br Med J 1999: 918:96-100.

Berga SL, Marcus MD, Loucks TL, Hlastala S, Ringham R, Krohn MA. Recovery of ovarian activity in women with functional hypothalamic amenorrhea who were treated with cognitive behavioral therapy. Fertil Steril 2003; 80:976-981.

Berlex Laboratories, Inc. YASMIN prescribing information: Physician Labeling and Patient Instructions; June, 2001.

Bjarnadottir R, Tuppurainen M, Killick S. Comparison of cycle control with a combined contraceptive vaginal ring and oral levonorgestrel/ethinyl estradiol. American Journal of Obstetrics and Gynecology. March 2002;186:389-95.

Brache V, Alvarez-Sanchez F, Faundes A, Tejada AS, Cochon L. Ovarian endocrine function through five years of continuous treatment with Norplant subdermal contraceptive implants. Contraception 1990;41:169.

Bradner, C.H., et al. Older, but Not Wiser: How Men Get Information About AIDS and ◀ Sexually Transmitted Diseases After High School. *Family Planning Perspectives* 2000; January/February.

Briggs GG, Freeman RK, Yaffe SJ. Drugs in Pregnancy and Lactation, Fifth edition. Lippincott Williams & Wilkins, Philadelphia. 1998.

Canto-DeCetina TEC, Canto P, Luna MO. Effect of counseling to improve compliance in Mexican women receiving depot-medroxyprogesterone acetate. Contraception 63; 2001: 143-146.

Cates W Jr., Steiner MJ. Dual protection against unintended pregnancy and sexually transmitted infections: What is the best contraceptive approach? Sex Transm Dis 2002;29:168-174.

Centers for Disease Control and Prevention. 1998 Guidelines for treatment of sexually transmitted diseases. MMWR 1998:47(No. RR-1).

Centers for Disease Control Cancer and Steroid Hormone Study. Long-term oral contraceptive use and the risk of breast cancer. JAMA. 1983; 249:1591-1595.

Colditz GA, Rosner BA, et al. Risk factors for breast cancer according to family history of breast cancer. J Natl Cancer Inst. 1996;88:365-371.

Collaborative Group on Hormonal Factors in Breast Cancer. Breast cancer and hormonal contraceptives: collaborative reanalysis of individual data on 53,297 women with breast cancer and 100,239 women without breast cancer from epidemiological studies. Lancet 1996; 347:1713-1727.

Coutinho EM with Segal SJ. Is Menstruation Obsolete? Oxford University Press; Oxford; New York; 1999.

Creinin MD, Burke AE. Methotrexate and misoprostol for early abortion: a multicenter trial. Acceptablity. Contraception 1996;54:19-22.

Creinin MD, Vittinghoff E, Schaff E, Klaisle C, Darney PD, Dean C. Medical abortion with oral methotrexate and vaginal misoprostol. Obstet Gynecol 1997;90:611-5.

Cromer BA, Lazebnik MD, Rome E et al. Double-blind controlled trial of estrogen ◄ supplementation in adolescent girls who receive depot medroxyprogesterone acetate for contraception. Am Jour Obstet Gynec 2005; 192:41-47.

Croxatto HB, Diaz S, Pavez M, et al. Plasma progesterone levels during long-term treatment with levonorgestrel silastic implants. Acta Endocrinol 1982;101:307-11.

Curtis et al. Contraception for Women in Selected Circumstances. Obstetrics and Gynecology, June 2002; 99 (6):1100-1112

Cundy T, Evans M, Roberts H, Wattie D, Ames R, Reid IR. Bone density in women receiving depot medroxyprogesterone acetate for contraception. BMJ 1991; 303: 13-16.

Davis KR, Weller SC. The effectiveness of condoms in reducing heterosexual transmission of HIV. Fam Plann Perspect 1999;31(6):272-279.

de Abood M, de Castillo 2, Guerrero E, Espino M, Austin KL. Effect of Depo-Provera or Microgynon in the painful crises of sickle-cell anemia patients. Contraception 56; 1997:313.

Diaz J, Bahamondes L, Monteiro I, Peta C, Hildalgo MM, Arce XE. Acceptability and performance of the levonorgestrel-releasing intrauterine system (Mirena) in Campinas, Brazil. Contraception 2000; 62: 59-61.

Dieben T, Roumen F, Apter D. Efficacy, cycle control, and user acceptability of a novel combined contraceptive vaginal ring. Obstetrics and Gynecology. Sept 2002; 100:585-93.

Edwards, S.R. The role of men in contraceptive decision-making: Current knowledge and ◄ future implications. *Family Planning Perspectives* 1994; March/April.

Farley TM, Rosenberg MS, Rowe PJ, Chen SH, Meirck O. Intrauterine devices and pelvic inflammatory disease: an international perspective. Lancet 1992; 339: 785-88.

Feldblum PJ, Morrison CS, Roddy RE, Cates W Jr. The effectiveness of barrier methods of contraception in preventing the spread of HIV. AIDS 1995;9 (suppl A):585-93.

Finer LB, Henshaw SK. Abortion incidence and service in the United States in 2000. Perspectives on Sexual and Reproductive Health 2003; 35(1): 6-15.

Ford K, Labbok M. Contraceptive use during lactation in the United States: an update. American Institute of Public Health 1987; 77: 79-81.

Forrest JD. U.S. women's perceptions of and attitudes about the IUD. Obstet Gynecol Surv. 1996; 31:S30-34

Fraser SI, Affandi B, Croxatto HB, et al. Norplant consensus statement and background paper. Turku, Finland: Leiras Oy International, 1997.

Frezieres RG, Walsh TL, Nelson AL, Clark VA, Coulson AH: Breakage and acceptability of a polyurethane condom: A randomized controlled study. Fam Plann Perspect 1998;30;73-8.

Glasier AF et al. Contraception 2003; 67:1-8.

Goldstein M, Girardi S. Vasectomy and vasectomy reversal. Curr Thera Endocrinol Metab 1997;6:371-80.

Grabrick DH, Hartmann LC, Cerhan FR, Vierkant RA, Therneau TM, et al. Risk of Breast Cancer with Oral Contraceptive Use in Women With a Family History of Breast Cancer. JAMA; 284:1791-1798.

Gray RH, Campbell OM, Zacur H, Labbok MH, MacRae SL. Postpartum return of ovarian activity in non-breastfeeding women monitored by urinary assays. J Clin Endocrinol Metab 1987;64:645-50.

Grimes DA. Health benefits of oral contraception: update on endometrial cancer prevention. The Contraception Report 2001;12(3):4-7.

Grimes DA. Modern IUDs: an update. The Contraception Report; November, 1998.

Grimes DA. Should first-time OC users be screened for genetic thrombophilia? The Contraception Report; 10:1, p.p. 9-11; March 1999.

Grimes DA. Transdermal contraceptive patch awaiting US approval. The Contraception Report; 12(4):12-14.

Grimes DA. IN Hatcher. Contraceptive Technology, 18th Ed. Intrauterine Devices (IUDS).

Guillebaud J. Contraception, your questions answered, 3rd edition. London, Churchill Livingstone, 1999.

Guillebaud J. Personal communication; October 14, 2001.

Hafner DW, Schwartz P. What I've Learned about Sex. A Perigee Book: New York: The Berkeley Publishing Group, 1998.

Hakim-Elahi E, Tovell HMM, Burnhill MS. Complications of first-trimester abortion: a report of 170,000 cases. Obstet Gynecol 1990;76:129.

Hall PE. New once-a-month injectable contraceptives, with particular reference to Cyclofem/ Cyclo-Provera. Int. J Gynaecol Obstet 1998; 62: S43-S56.

Hausknecht R. Mifepristone and misoprostol for early medical abortion: 18 months experience in the United States. Contraception 2003; 67:463-465.

Haws, J.M., et al. Clinical Practice of vasectomies in the United States in 1995. *Urology* 1998; October.

Henshaw SK. Unintended pregnancy in the United States. Fam Plann Perspect 1998;30:24-9, 46.

Hatcher RA, Trussell J, Stewart F, Cates W Jr, Stewart GK, Guest F, Kowal D. *Contraceptive Technology*, 17th ed. New York NY, Ardent Media, 1998

Hilgers, T.W., Abraham, G.E., and Cavanagh, D. (1978), "Natural Family Planning. I. The Peak Symptom and Estimated Time of Ovulation", *Obstetrics and Gynecology* 52(5): 575-582.

Hogue CJR, Cates W Jr, Tietze C. The effects of induced abortion on subsequent reproduction. The Johns Hopkins University School of Hygiene and Public Health. Epidemiol Rev 1982;4:66

International Planned Parenthood Federation Handbook 1997.

Jain J, Jakimiuk AJ, Bode FR, Ross D, Kaunitz AM. Contraceptive efficacy and safety ← of DMPA-SC. Contraception 2004; 70:269-275.

Jamieson DJ, Costello C, Trussell J, Hillis SP, Marckbanks PA, Peterson HB. The risk of ← pregnancy after vasectomy. Obstetrics and Gynecology 2004; 103: 848-850.

Jones RK, Dorroch JE, Henshaw SK. Patterns with socioeconomic characterics of women obtaining abortions in 2000-2001. Perspectives in Sexual and Reproductive Health 2002;34:226-235.

Kaunitz AM. personal communications; December 28, 1998 and February 24, 1999.

Kaunitz AM, Garceau RJ, Cromie MA. Comparative safety, efficacy, and cycle control of Lunelle monthly contraceptive injection (medroxyprogesterone acetate and estradiol cypionate injectable suspension) and Ortho-Novum 7/7/7 oral contraceptive (norethindrone/ethinyl estradiol triphasic). Contraception 1999; 60(4):179-187.

Kennedy KI, Trussell J. Postpartum contraception and lactation. IN Hatcher RA, Trussell J, Stewart F et al: Contraceptive Technology, 17th ed.; New York: Ardent Media Inc; 1998: 592-4. [The same data are presented in the Family Health International Module for the teaching of Lactational Amenorrhea]

Kjos SL, Peters RK, Xiang A, Duncan T, Schaefer U, Buchanan TA. Contraception and the risk of type 2 diabetes mellitus in Latina women with prior gestational diabetes mellitus. JAMA 1998; 280: 533-38.

Klavon SL, Grubb G. Insertion site complications during the first year of Norplant use. Contraception 1990;41:27.

Krattenmacher R. Drospirenone: pharmacology and pharmacokinetics of a unique progestogen. Contraception 2000; 62:29-38.

Kuyoh MA, Toroitich-Ruto C, Grimes DA, et al. Sponge versus diaphragm for ← contraception: a Cochrane review. Contraception 2003; 67(1):15-18.

Kwiecien M et al. Contraception 2003; 67:9-13.

Lipnick RJ, Buring JE, Hennekens CH, et al. Oral contraceptives and breast cancer: a prospective cohort study. JAMA. 1986; 255:58-61.

Lippes J (Guest Editor). Quinacrine sterilization: reports on 40,252 cases. Intl J of Gynec & Obstet Volume 83, supl 2, October 2003.

Marcell, A.V., et al. Where Does Reproductive Health Fit Into the Lives of Adolescent ← Males? Perspectives of Sexual and Reproductive Health 2003; 35(4):180-186.

Marguilies R, Miller L. Increased depot medroxyprogesterone acetate use increases family planning program pharmaceutical supply costs. Contraception 2001 (63):147-149.

Michaelson, M.D., Oh, W.K. Epidemiology of and risk factors for testicular cancer. ← Available from http://www.utdol.com [Accessed 10 October 2004]

Miller L, Grice J. Intradermal proximal field block: an innovative anesthetic technique for levonorgestrel implant removal. Obstet Gynecol 1998;91:294-297.

Monteiro I, Bahamondes L, Diaz J, Perotti M, Petta C. Therapeutic use of levonorgestrel-releasing intrauterine systems in women with menorrhagia: a pilot study. Contraception 65; 2002; 325-328.

Mulders TMT, Dieben TOM. Use of the novel combined contraceptive vaginal ring NuvaRing for ovulation inhibition. Fertility and Sterility 2001; 75:865-870.

Murray PP, Stadel BV, Schlesselman JJ. Oral contraceptive use in women with a family history of breast cancer. Obstet Gynecol. 1989; 73:977-983.

Narod ST. The Hereditary Ovarian Cancer Clinical Study Group. Oral contraceptives and the risk of hereditary ovarian cancer. N Engl J Med 1998;339;424-8.

Narod ST. et al. Lancet 357 [9267]: 1467-70, 2001.

Ness RB, Grisso JA, Klapper J, et al. Risk of ovarian cancer in relation to estrogen and progestin dose and use characteristics of oral contraceptives. Am J Epidemiol 2000;152:233-241.

Ness, R.B., et al. Do men become infertile after having sexually transmitted urethritis? An epidemiologic examination. *Fertility and Sterility* 1997; 68(2):205-213. ◄

O'Hanley K, Huber DH. Postpartum IUDs: keys for success. Contraception 1992; 45: 351-361.

Peipert JF, Gutman J. Oral contraceptive risk assessment: a survey of 247 educated women. Obstet Gynecol 1993;82:112-7.

Peterson HB, Jeng G, Folger SG et al for the U.S. Collaborative Review of Sterilization Working Group. N Engl J Med 2000; 343:1681-7.

Peterson HB, Pollack AE, Warshaw JS. Tubal sterilization. In: Rock JA, Thompson JD, eds. TeLinde's Operative Gynecology. 8th ed. Philadelphia: Lippincott-Raven, 1997:541-5.

Pinkerton SD, Abramson PR. Effectiveness of condoms in preventing HIV transmission. Soc Sci Med 1997 May; 44(9):1303-1312.

Plichta, S.B., et al. Partner-specific condom use among adolescent women clients of a ◄ amily planning clinic. *Journal of Adolescent Health* 1992; 13(6):506-511.

Polaneczky M, Guarnaccia, Alon J, Wiley J. Early experience with the contraceptive use of depot medroxyprogesterone acetate in an inner-city clinic population. Family Planning Perspectives 1996; 28: 174-178.

Porter, L.E., Ku, L. Use of reproductive health services among young men, 1995. ◄ *Journal of Adolescent Health* 1995; 27(3):186-194.

Raudaskoski TH, Lahti EI, Kauppila AJ, Apaja-Sarkkinen MA, Laatikainen TJ. Transdermal estrogen with a levonorgestrel-releasing intrauterine device for climacteric complaints: clinical and endometrial responses. Am J Obstet Gynecol 1995;172:114-9.

Redmond G, Godwin AJ, Olson W, Lippman JS. Use of placebo controls in an oral contraceptive trial: methodological issues and adverse event incidence. Contraception 1999;60:81-5.

Ropes ASW. Menstrual suppression survey, 2002.

Roumen FJ, Apter D, Mulders TM, et al. Efficacy, tolerability and acceptability of a novel contraceptive vaginal ring releasing etonogestrel and ethinyl estradiol. Hum Reprod 2001;16:469-475.

Schwallie PC, Assenzo JR. Contraceptive use-efficacy study initializing medroxy-progesterone acetate administered as an intramuscular injection once every 90 days. Fertil Steril 1973; 24(5):331-339.

Segal SJ. Is menstration obsolete? Lecture in Atlanta, Georgia. November 1, 2001.

Shelton JD. Repeat emergency contraception: facing our fears. Contraception 66;2002:15-17.

Silvestre L, Dubois C, Renault M, Rezvani Y, Baulieu E, Ullmann A. Voluntary interruption of pregnancy with mifepristone (RU-486) and a prostaglandin analogue. N Engl J Med 1990; 322:645-8.

Sivin I, Stern J et al. Prolonged intrauterine contraception: a seven-year randomized study of the levonorgestrel 20 mcg/day (LNG 20) and the Copper T 380Ag IUDs. Contraception 1991; 44:473-80

Shulman LP, Oleen-Burkey M, Willke RJ. Patient acceptability and satisfaction with Lunelle monthly contraceptive injection (medroxyprogesterone acetate and estradiol cipionate injectable suspension). Contraception 1999;60(4):215-222.

Smith TW. Personal communication to James Trussell. December 13, 1993.

Sonfield, A. Looking at Men's Sexual and Reproductive Health Needs. *The Guttmacher Report on Public Policy* 2002; November. ◄

Sonfield, A. Meeting the Sexual and Reproductive Health Needs of Men Worldwide. *The Guttmacher Report on Public Policy* 2004; March. ◄

Speroff PD. A Clinical Guide for Contraception. Third Edition. Lippincott Williams & Wilkins; Philadelphia; 2001.

Speroff L, Glass RH, Kase NG. Clinical Gynecologic Endocrinology and Infertility. Sixth Edition. 1999; Lipincott Williams & Wilkins; Baltimore, Maryland.

Speroff L. The perimenospausal transition: maximizing preventive health care. In: Mooney B, Daughtery J, eds. Midlife Women's Health Sourcebook. Atlanta: American Health Consultants, 1995.

Steiner MJ. Cates W Jr, Warner L. The real problems with male condoms is nonuse. Sex Trans Dis 1999;26(8):459-61.

Stencheuer MA. Comprehensive Gynecology Fourth Edition. Mosby. 2001

Stewart FH, Harper CC, Ellertson CE, Grimes DA, Sawyer GF, Trussell J. Clinical breast and pelvic examination requirements for hormonal contraception: Current practice vs. evidence. JAMA 2001;285:2232-2239.

Sulak PJ et al. Am J Obstet Gynecol 2002; 186:1142-1149.

Sulak PJ et al. Obstet Gynecol 2000; 95:261-266.

Task Force on Postovulatory Methods of Fertility Regulation. Randomized controlled trial of levonorgestrel versus the Yuzpe regimen of combined oral contraceptives for emergency contraception. Lancet 1998;352:420-33.

The Alan Guttmacher Institute. Sex and America's Teenagers. New York and Washington: 1994.

The Hereditary Ovarian Cancer Clinical Study Group. Oral contraceptives and the risk of hereditary ovarian cancer. N Engl J Med 1998;339;424-8.

Truitt ST, Fraser AB, Grimes DA, Gallo MF, Schulz KF. Hormonal contraception during lactation: a systematic reivew of randomized controlled trials. Contraception 2003; 68:233-8.

Trussell J, Leveque JA, Koenig JD, London R, Borden S, Henneberry J, LaGuardia KD, Stewart F, Wilson TG, Wysocki S, Strauss M. The economic value of contraception: a comparison of 15 methods. Am J Public Health 1995;85:494-503.

Trussell J, Stewart F, Guest F, Hatcher RA. Emergency contraceptive pills: a simple proposal to reduce unintended pregnancies. Fam Plann Perspect 1992;24:269-73.

Tschugguel W, Berga SL. Treatment of functional hypothalamic amenorrhea with hypnotherapy. Fertil Steril. 2003; 80:982-985.

Valle RF, Carignan CS, Wright TC, et al. Tissue response to STOP microcoil transcervical permanent contraceptive device: results from a prehysterectomy study. Fertil Steril 2001; 76:974.

Vercellini P et al. Fertil Steril 2003; 80:560-63.

Von Hertzen H, Piaggio G, Ding J et al. Low dose Mifepristone and two regimens of levonorgestrel for emergency contraception: a WHO multicentre randomised trial. Lancet 2002; 360: 1803-10.

Walsh T, Grimes D, Frezieres R, Nelson A, Bernstein L, Coulson A, Bernstein G. Randomized controlled trial of prophylactic antibiotics before insertion of intrauterine devices. *Lancet* 1998:351;1005-1008.

Warner DL, Hatcher RA, Boles J, Goldsmith J. Practices and patterns of condom usage for prevention of infection and pregnancy among male university students (Session PS-12). Proceeding of the Eleventh Annual National Preventive Medicine Meeting. March 1994.

Warner L, Hatcher RA, Steiner MJ. Male Condoms. IN Hatcher RA et al. Contraceptive Technology 18th Edition. 2004.

Weidner, W., et al. Relevance of male accessory gland infection for subsequent fertility ← with special focus on prostatitis. *Human Reproduction Update* 1999; 5(5):421-432.

Westoff C, Kerns J, Morroni C, Cushman LF, Tiezzi L, Murphy PA. Quick Start: a novel contraceptive initiation method. Contraception 66; 2002:141-145.

White MK, Ory HW, Rooks JB, Rochat RW. Intrauterine device termination rates and menstrual cycle day of insertion. Obstet Gynecol 1980; 55:220-4.

Willett WC, Green A, Stampfer MJ, Speizer FE, Colditz GA, Rosner B, Monson RR, Stason W, Hennekens CH. Relative and absolute risks of coronary heart disease among women who smoke cigarettes. New Eng J Med 317:1303, 1987.

World Health Organization, Department of Reproductive Health and Research. Improving Access to Quality Care in Family Planning: Medical Eligibility Criteria for Contraceptive Use. Second Edition. Geneva. 2000.

World Health Organization. WHO Taskforce Postovulatory Methods of Fertility Regulation. Lancet Aug 8, 1998.

Writing Group for the Women's Health Initiative. Risks and benefits of estrogen plus progestin in healthy postmenopausal women. JAMA 2002; 288: 321-333.

Zieman M, Guillebaud J, Weisberg E, Shangold G, Fisher A, Creasy G. Integrated summary of contraceptive efficacy with the Ortho Evra transdermal system. Fertility and Sterility Supplement; September, 2001. S19

IMPORTANT WEBSITES

TOPIC	WEBSITE
Abortion	www.prochoice.org
	www.ipas.org ←
Adolescent Reproductive Health	www.teenpregnancy.org
	www.ama-assn.org/adolhlth/adolhlth.htm
	www.advocatesforyouth.org
Contraception	www.conrad.org
	www.who.int (World Health Organization Precautions)
	www.contraceptiononline.org/contrareport
	www.managingcontraception.com
	www.ippfwhr.org
	www.plannedparenthood.org
	www.reproline.jhu.edu
	www.engenderhealth.org ←
Counseling	www.gmhc.org
Education	www.siecus.org
	www.cdc.gov
Emergency Contraception	www.not-2-late.com or http://ec.princeton.edu
HIV/AIDS/STIs	www.CritPath.Org/aric
	www.cdc.gov/hiv
	www.cdc.gov/nchstp/dstd/dstdp.htm
Managing Contraception	www.managingcontraception.com
Menopause	www.menopause.org
	www.osteo.org
Natural Family Planning	www.canfp.org
(Fertility Awareness)	www.irh.org ←
	www.ccli.org
Population Organizations	www.popcouncil.org
	www.prb.org
	www.undp.org/popin/infoserv.htm
	www.population.org/homepage.htm
Professional Organizations	www.acog.org
	www.arhp.org
	www.fda.gov
	www.fhi.org
	www.jsi.com
	www.NPWH.org
	www.pathfind.org
	www.plannedparenthood.org
	www.who.int
Reproductive Health Research	www.guttmacher.org ←
	www.fhi.org
	www.ipm.microbicides.org ←

SPANISH/ENGLISH TRANSLATIONS

SPANISH/ESPAÑOL	ENGLISH/INGLES
• Abstinencia	• Abstinence
• Amamantar a Su Bebe	• Breast-feeding
• Tapa Cervical	• Cervical Cap
• Retraer el pene antes de eyacular	• Coitus Interruptus (Withdrawal)
• Injecciones Combinadas	• Combined Injectables
• La Pildora	• Combined Oral Contraceptives (COCs)
• Condones parce hombres	• Condoms for Men
• Condones para Mujeres	• Condoms for Women
• La "T" o Dispositivo do Cobre	• Copper T 380-A
• Injecciones de Depo-Provera	• Depo-Provera
• El Diafragma	• Diaphragm
• Contraceptivo de Emergencia	• Emergency Contraception
• Consciente Sobre Metodos de Fertilidad	• Fertility Awareness Methods
• Espuma Contraceptiva	• Foam
• Metodos para el Futuro	• Future Methods
• Dispositivos	• IUDs
• Gelatina Anticonceptiva	• Jellies
• El Dispositivo de "Levo Norgestrel"	• Levonorgestrel IUD
• Implantes de NORPLANT	• Norplant Implant
• El Dispositivo de "Progestasert"	• Progestasert IUD
• Contraceptives de Progesterona Solamente	• Progestin-Only Contraceptives
• Pildoras de Progesterona Solamente	• Progestin-Only Pills (POPs)
• RU-486 (Mifepristone)	• RU-486 (Mifepristone)
• Espermicidas	• Spermicides
• Ligadura o Estirilizacion de las Trompas	• Tubal Sterilization
• Tela Anticonceptiva	• Vaginal contraceptive film
• Vasectomia	• Vasectomy
• Todos los dispositivos	• All other IUDs at this time

<u>**NOTE:**</u> **Final pages of Appendix (A18 - A26) are at very end of book**

A Personal
Guide to Contraception
la planificacion familiar
Order in Spanish online at:
www.managingcontraception.com

INDEX

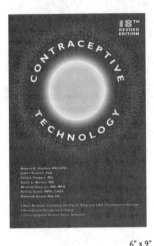

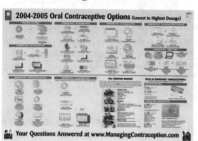
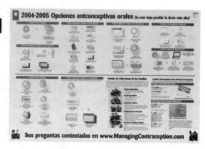

Contraceptive Choices

The perfect set of contraceptive descriptions to give to patients with all the current methods explained in detail, including advantages and disadvantages. Developed by Dr. Robert A. Hatcher.

Code #5200

(minimum 10 copies) $13.00;
11-25 ($1.25 ea.); 26-50 ($1.20 ea.);
over 50 ($1.10 ea.) or 100 for $99.95

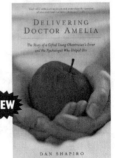

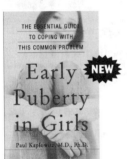

Early Puberty in Girls

The definitive book about early puberty in girls – what it is, how it happens, when to be concerned, and how it should be treated.

Code #5400 $13.95 each

Delivering Doctor Amelia

The story of a gifted young obstetrician's error and the psychologist who helped her. Explores with startling depth the question of who shall heal the fallen physician.

Code #5300 $13.00 each

Order online: www.ManagingContraception.com

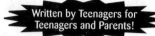
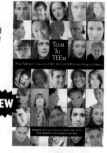
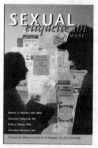
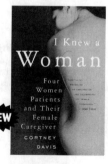

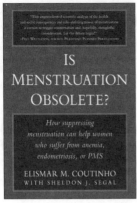

Is Menstruation Obsolete?

Is Menstruation Obsolete? argues that regular monthly bleeding is not the natural state of women and that it actually places them at risk of several medical conditions of varying severity.

Code #4016

$24.00 each (Hardcover)

Devices and Desires: A History of Contraceptives in America

Andrea Tone's informative recount of the contraceptive culture in America, beginning with its significance in the late 19th century and concluding with issues faced in the last two decades.

Code #4015

$30.00 each (Hardcover)

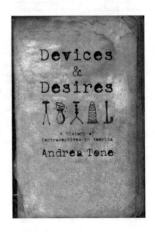

ORDER FORM

Call to order or for Customer Service:

706-265-7435, ext. 10

BY MAIL:
Bridging the Gap
P.O. Box 888
Dawsonville. GA 30534

BY FAX:
706-265-6009

ONLINE:
www.ManagingContraception.com
24 Hours a Day. Enjoy Shopping!

ORDERED BY

Name _____ Title _____

Organization _____

Address _____

City _____ State _____ Zip _____

E-mail Address _____

Phone _____ Fax _____

SHIP TO (Only if different from Ordered By)

Name _____ Title _____

Organization _____

Address _____

City _____ State _____ Zip _____

Item Code #	Description	Qty.	Price Ea.	Item Total
_____	_____	_____	_____	_____
_____	_____	_____	_____	_____
_____	_____	_____	_____	_____
_____	_____	_____	_____	_____
_____	_____	_____	_____	_____
_____	_____	_____	_____	_____
_____	_____	_____	_____	_____
_____	_____	_____	_____	_____
_____	_____	_____	_____	_____
_____	_____	_____	_____	_____
_____	_____	_____	_____	_____

SUBTOTAL _____

Payment Method:

☐ MasterCard ☐ VISA ☐ Discover

☐ American Express ☐ Personal Check

☐ Purchase Order #_____
(For Organizations Only)

Credit Card Number:

_____

Valid through _____

Signature _____

Merchandise Subtotal:	_____
GA Sales Tax (7%)	_____
Subtotal	_____
*Shipping (Add 15%)	_____
Handling	**$1.00**
TOTAL (US funds only)	_____

Phone (required) _____

*International Shipping: Alaska, Hawaii, Puerto Rico, Canada and all others not in the
48 contiguous United States, call for shipping prices.

Prices valid until superceded by subsequent publication.

Thank You for Your Order!

Your contraceptive questions answered at
www.ManagingContraception.com

The mission of Bridging The Gap Foundation is to improve reproductive health and contraceptive decision-making of women and men by providing up-to-date educational resources to the physicians, nurses and public health leaders of tomorrow.

Our vision is to provide educational resources to the health care providers of tomorrow to help ensure informed choices, better service, access, happier and more successful contraceptors, competent clinicians, fewer unintended pregnancies and disease prevention.

www.bridgingthegapfoundation.org

 Order online: www.ManagingContraception.com

COLOR PHOTOS

of Combined and Progestin-Only Oral Contraceptives
www.managingcontraception.com

The TEN color pages of pills are organized as follows:

Color photos of pills from lowest to highest estrogen dose..........A19-A28

- Progestin-only pills with **no estrogen**: Micronor, NOR-QD, and Ovrette
- Lowest estrogen pills with **20 micrograms** of the estrogen, ethinyl estradiol: Alesse, Levlite, LoEstrin 1/20, and Mircette
- All of the 25-, **30- and 35-microgram** pills (all ethinyl estradiol)
- All of the **phasic** pills
- Highest estrogen pills, with **50 micrograms** of estrogen (ethinyl estradiol OR mestranol). Mestranol is converted in the body to ethinyl estradiol; 50 mcg of mestranol is equivalent to 35 mcg of ethinyl estradiol

There are prominent horizontal or vertical parallel lines ("equal signs") between pills which are pharmacologically exactly the same. The color and packaging of pills dispensed in clinics may differ from pills in pharmacies.

Pill Warning Signals..A29
The "ACHES" method of teaching women on pills what to watch out for and the problems a clinician or counselor should think about if one of these symptoms develops.

Pills you can prescribe as emergency contraceptive pills...............A30

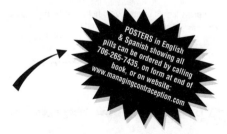

POSTERS in English & Spanish showing all pills can be ordered by calling 706-265-7435, on form at end of book, or on website: www.managingcontraception.com

**MICRONOR® TABLETS
28-DAY REGIMEN**
(0.35 mg norethindrone) (lime green)
Ortho-McNeil

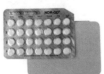

NOR-QD® TABLETS
(0.35 mg norethindrone) (yellow)
Watson

NORA BE
(0.35 mg norethindrone)
(yellow)
Watson

ERRIN
(0.35 mg norethindrone) (yellow)
Barr

JOLIVETTE
(0.35 mg norethindrone) (lime green)
Watson

CAMILA
(0.35 mg norethindrone) (light pink)

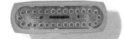

OVRETTE® TABLETS
(0.075 mg norgestrel) (yellow)
Wyeth

A19

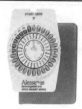

ALESSE - 28 TABLETS
(active pills pink)
Wyeth

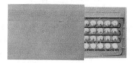

LEVLITE™ - 28 TABLETS
(0.1 mg levonorgestrel/20 mcg ethinyl estradiol)
(active pills pink)
Berlex

AVIANE
(0.1 mg levonorgestrel/20 mcg ethinyl estradiol)
(active pills orange)
Barr

LESSINA-28
(0.1 mg levonorgestrel/20 mcg ethinyl estradiol)
(active pills pink)

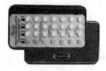

MIRCETTE - 28 TABLETS
(0.15 mg desogestrel/ 20 mcg ethinyl estradiol X 21 (white)/
placebo X 2 (green)/10 mcg ethinyl estradiol X 5 (yellow)
Organon

KARIVA 28
(0.15 mg desogestrel/ 20 mcg ethinyl estradiol X 21 (white)/
placebo X 2 (green)/10 mcg ethinyl estradiol X 5 (light blue)
Barr

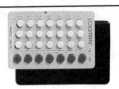

LOESTRIN® FE 1/20
(1 mg norethindrone acetate/20 mcg ethinyl
estradiol/75 mg ferrous fumarate [7d])
(active pills white)
Barr

MICROGESTIN FE 1/20
(1 mg norethindrone acetate/20 mcg ethinyl
estradiol/75 mg ferrous fumarate [7d])
Watson

JUNEL FE 1/20
(1 mg norethindrone acetate/20 mcg ethinyl
estradiol/75 mg ferrous fumarate [7d])
(active pills yellow)
Barr

LEVLEN® 28 TABLETS
(0.15 mg levonorgestrel/30 mcg ethinyl estradiol)
(active pills light orange)
Berlex

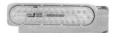

NORDETTE®-28 TABLETS
(0.15 mg levonorgestrel/30 mcg ethinyl estradiol)
(active pills light orange)
Monarch

LEVORA TABLETS
(0.15 mg levonorgestrel/30 mcg ethinyl estradiol)
(active pills white)
Watson

PORTIA 28
(0.15 mg levonorgestrel/30 mcg ethinyl estradiol)
(active pills pink)
Barr

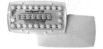

SEASONALE
(0.15 mg levonorgestrel/30 mcg ethinyl estradiol)
84 active pills followed by 7 placebo pills

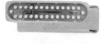

LO/OVRAL®-28 TABLETS
(0.3 mg norgestrel/30 mcg ethinyl estradiol)
(active pills white)
Wyeth

LOW-OGESTREL - 28
(0.3 mg norgestrel/30 mcg ethinyl estradiol)
(active pills white)
Watson

CRYSELLE
(0.3 mg norgestrel/30 mcg ethinyl estradiol)
(active pills white)
Barr

DESOGEN® 28 TABLETS
(0.15 mg desogestrel/30 mcg ethinyl estradiol)
(active pills white)
Organon

**ORTHO-CEPT® TABLETS
28-DAY REGIMEN**
(0.15 mg desogestrel/30 mcg ethinyl estradiol)
(active pills orange)
Ortho-McNeil

APRI
(0.15 mg
(active pills rose)
Barr

LOESTRIN® 21 1.5/30 (With & Without Fe)
(1.5 mg norethindrone acetate/ 30 mcg ethinyl estradiol)
(active pills green)
Barr

MICROGESTIN 1.5/30 (With & Without Fe)
Watson

JUNEL Fe 1.5/30
(active pills pink)
Barr

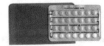

YASMIN 28 TABLETS
(3.0 mg drospirenone/30 mcg ethinyl estradiol)
(active pills yellow)
Berlex

COMBINED PILLS - 35 microgram PILLS

OVCON® 35 28-DAY
(0.4 mg norethindrone/35 mcg ethinyl estradiol)
(active pills peach)
Warner-Chilcott
Now there is a chewable Ovcon-35 pill!

ORTHO-CYCLEN®
28 TABLETS
(0.25 mg norgestimate/35 mcg ethinyl estradiol)
(active pills blue)
Ortho-McNeil

MONONESESSA
(0.25 mg norgestimate/35 mcg ethinyl estradiol)
Watson

SPRINTEC
(0.25 mg norgestimate/35 mcg ethinyl estradiol)
(active pills blue)
Barr

BREVICON®
28-DAY TABLETS
(0.5 mg norethindrone/35 mcg ethinyl estradiol)
(active pills blue)
Watson

MODICON® TABLETS
28-DAY REGIMEN
(0.5 mg norethindrone/35 mcg ethinyl estradiol)
(active pills white)
Ortho-McNeil

NORTREL
(0.5 mg norethindrone/35 mcg ethinyl estradiol)
Barr

NECON 0.5/35
(0.5 mg norethindrone/35 mcg ethinyl estradiol)
Watson

DEMULEN® 1/35-28
(1 mg ethynodiol diacetate/35 mcg ethinyl estradiol)
(active pills white)
Pharmacia

ZOVIA® 1/35E–28
(1 mg ethynodiol diacetate/35 mcg ethinyl estradiol)
(active pills light pink)
Watson

**ORTHO-NOVUM® 1/35
28 TABLETS**
(1 mg norethindrone/35 mcg ethinyl estradiol)
(active pills peach)
Ortho-McNeil

NORINYL® 1+35 28-DAY TABLETS
(1 mg norethindrone/35 mcg ethinyl estradiol)
(active pills yellow-green)
Watson

NECON 1/35-28
(1 mg norethindrone/35 mcg ethinyl estradiol)
(active pills dark yellow)
Watson

NORTREL
(1 mg norethindrone/35 mcg ethinyl estradiol)
Barr

ORTHO TRI-CYCLEN® LO - 28 TABLETS
(norgestimate/ethinyl estradiol)
0.18 mg/25 mcg (7d) (white),
0.215 mg/25 mcg (7d) (light blue),
0.25 mg/25 mcg (7d) (dark blue)
remaining 7 placebo pills are green
Ortho-McNeil

TRINESSA
Watson

VELIVET
(desogestrel/ethinyl estradiol–triphasic regimen)
0.1 mg/25 mcg (7d) (beige)
0.125 mg/25 mcg (7d) (orange)
0.150 mg/25 mcg (7d) (pink)
Barr

CYCLESSA
(desogestrel/ethinyl estradiol–triphasic regimen)
0.1 mg/25 mcg (7d) (light yellow)
0.125 mg/25 mcg (7d) (orange)
0.150 mg/25 mcg (7d) (red)
Organon

TRIVORA®
(levonorgestrel/ethinyl estradiol–triphasic regimen)
0.050 mg/30 mcg (6d), 0.075 mg/40 mcg (5d),
0.125 mg/30 mcg (10d) (pink)
Watson

TRIPHASIL®-28 TABLETS
(levonorgestrel/ethinyl estradiol–triphasic regimen)
0.050 mg/30 mcg (6d) (brown),
0.075 mg/40 mcg (5d) (white),
0.125 mg/30 mcg (10d) (light yellow)
Wyeth-Ayerst

TRI-LEVLEN® 28 TABLETS
(levonorgestrel/ethinyl estradiol–triphasic regimen)
0.050 mg/30 mcg (6d) (brown),
0.075 mg/40 mcg (5d) (white),
0.125 mg/30 mcg (10d) (light yellow)
Berlex

ENPRESSE
(levonorgestrel/ethinyl estradiol–triphasic regimen)
0.050 mg/30 mcg (6d) (pink),
0.075 mg/40 mcg (5d) (white),
0.125 mg/30 mcg (10d) (orange)
Barr

ORTHO-NOVUM® 10/11 28 TABLETS
(norethindrone/ethinyl estradiol)
0.5 mg/35 mcg (10d) (white),
1 mg/35 mcg (11d) (peach)
Ortho-McNeil

NECON 10/11
(norethindrone/ethinyl estradiol)
0.5 mg/35 mcg (10d) (white),
1 mg/35 mcg (11d) (peach)
Watson

TRI-NORINYL® 28-DAY TABLETS
(norethindrone/ethinyl estradiol)
0.5 mg/35 mcg (7d) (blue),
1 mg/35 mcg (9d) (yellow-green),
0.5 mg/35 mcg (5d) (blue)
Watson

ORTHO TRI-CYCLEN® 28 TABLETS
(norgestimate/ethinyl estradiol)
0.18 mg/35 mcg (7d) (white),
0.215 mg/35 mcg (7d) (light blue),
0.25 mg/35 mcg (7d) (blue)
Ortho-McNeil

TRI-SPRINTEC 28
(norgestimate/ethinyl estradiol)
0.18 mg/35 mcg (7d) (gray),
0.215 mg/35 mcg (7d) (light blue),
0.25 mg/35 mcg (7d) (blue)
Barr

ORTHO-NOVUM® 7/7/7 28 TABLETS
(norethindrone/ethinyl estradiol)
0.5 mg/35 mcg (7d) (white),
0.75 mg/35 mcg (7d) (light peach),
1 mg/35 mcg (7d) (peach)
Ortho-McNeil

NORTREL 7/7/7
(norethindrone/ethinyl estradiol)
0.5 mg/35 mcg (7d) (yellow),
0.75 mg/35 mcg (7d) (blue),
1 mg/35 mcg (7d) (peach)
Barr

ESTROSTEP® FE 28 TABLETS
(norethindrone acetate/ethinyl estradiol)
1 mg/20 mcg (5d) (white triangular),
1 mg/30 mcg (7d) (white square),
1 mg/35 mcg (9d), 75 mg ferrous fumarate (7d)
(white round)
Warner-Chilcott

NECON 7/7/7
(norethindrone/ethinyl estradiol)
0.5 mg/35 mcg (7d) (yellow),
0.75 mg/35 mcg (7d) (blue),
1 mg/35 mcg (7d) (peach)
Watson

COMBINED PILLS - 50 microgram PILLS

Pills with 50 micrograms of mestranol are not as strong as pills with 50 micrograms of ethinyl estradiol

ORTHO-NOVUM® 1/50 28 TABLETS
(1 mg norethindrone/50 mcg mestranol)
(active pills yellow)
Ortho-McNeil

NECON 1/50
(1 mg norethindrone/50 mcg mestranol)
Watson

NORINYL 1/50
(1 mg norethindrone/50 mcg mestranol)
Watson

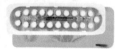

OVRAL - 21 TABLETS
(0.5 mg norgestrel/50 mcg ethinyl estradiol)
(active pills white)
Wyeth-Ayerst

OGESTREL
(0.5 mg norgestrel/50 mcg ethinyl estradiol)
Watson

OVCON® 50 28-DAY
(1 mg norethindrone/50 mcg ethinyl estradiol)
(active pills yellow)
Warner-Chilcott

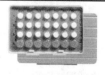

DEMULEN® 1/50-28
(1 mg ethynodiol diacetate/50 mcg ethinyl estradiol)
(active pills white)
Pharmacia

ZOVIA 1/50
(1 mg ethynodiol diacetate/50 mcg ethinyl estradiol)
Watson

PILL WARNING SIGNALS

Pills have been studied extensively and are very safe. However, very rarely pills lead to serious problems. Here are the warning signals to watch out for while using pills. These warning signals spell out the word **ACHES**. If you have one of these symptoms, it may or may not be related to pill use. You need to check with your clinician as soon as possible. The problems that could possibly be related to using pills are as follows:

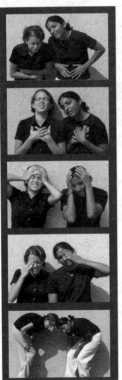

ABDOMINAL PAIN
- Blood clot in the pelvis or liver
- Gall bladder disease

CHEST PAIN
- Blood clot in the lungs
- Heart attack
- Angina (heart pain)

HEADACHES
- Stroke
- Migraine headache with neurological problems (blurred vision, spots, zigzag lines, weakness, difficulty speaking)
- New onset or worsening headache
- High blood pressure

EYE PROBLEMS
- Stroke
- Blurred vision, double vision, or loss of vision
- Migraine headache with neurological problems (blurred vision, spots, zigzag lines)
- Blood clots in the eyes
- Change in shape of cornea (contacts don't fit)

SEVERE LEG PAIN
- Inflammation and blood clots of a vein in the leg

You should also return to the office if you develop severe mood swings or depression, become jaundiced (yellow-colored skin), miss 2 periods or have signs of pregnancy.

PILLS AS EMERGENCY CONTRACEPTIVES:

2 Different Approaches: Progestin-Only Pills OR Combined Pills

PROGESTIN-ONLY PILLS

Plan B

1 + 1 pill **12 hours apart OR**
2 Plan B Pills *(white)* ASAP after
unprotected sex

20 + 20 pills **12 hours apart**

Ovrette *(yellow pills)*

(Plan B and Ovrette are NOT carried in all pharmacies.
Check in advance. Ask your pharmacy to carry Plan B

plan B™
(LEVONORGESTREL)

PLAN B

Antinausea meds <u>not</u> necessary

COMBINED ORAL CONTRACEPTIVES

2 + 2 pills **12 hours apart**

Ovral *(white pills)*
Preven *(blue pills)* (no longer marketed)
Ogestrel *(white pills)*
Zovia (   )

(Ogestrel, Zovia and Ovral are NOT
carried in all pharmacies. Check in
advance.)

4 + 4 pills **12 hours apart**

Lo-Ovral *(white pills)*, OR
Levlen *(light orange pills)* OR
Levora *(white pills)* OR
Low-Ogestrel *(white pills)* OR
Nordette *(light orange pills)* OR
Triphasil *(yellow pills)*, OR
Tri-Levlen *(yellow pills)* OR
Trivora *(pink pills)*

> Have your patient take
> antinausea medication an
> hour before the first dose if
> using any of the combined
> oral contraceptives as
> emergency contraception.
> This is <u>not</u> necessary if
> using Plan B.

5 + 5 pills **12 hours apart**

Alesse *(pink pills)* OR
Aviane *(orange pills)* OR
Lessina *(pink pills)* OR
Levlite *(pink pills)* OR
Enpresse *(orange pills)* OR
Portia *(pink pills)* OR
Seasonale *(pink pills)*